Involuntary childlessness affects an estimated 15% of the U.K. adult population but its personal and social effect is little understood. For those who are, or who realise they may be childless, this isolating experience is particularly exaggerated by a society geared towards parenting and children.

With the increasing difficulty in adoption and fostering, and recent developments in artificial insemination, test tube conception and surrogate mothering, there is a further emphasis for the childless to explore every possible medical solution. Greater hopes and expectations are raised, very often as the prelude to greater disappointments.

Until now little has been written about the emotional needs of the childless. Diane and Peter Houghton – themselves childless – have drawn on their personal experiences of tests, treatments, social prejudices and final readjustment to write this book. Peter Houghton originated the National Association for the Childless in 1976 which continues to serve an ever increasing need to counsel, console, help and advise the childless.

The authors' uniquely wide experience and humanity makes *Coping with Childlessness* essential reading, both for the childless and for those health professionals who need a full understanding of the experience of childlessness.

COPING WITH
CHILDLESSNESS

DIANE & PETER HOUGHTON

UNWIN PAPERBACKS

London   Sydney

First published in Great Britain by Allen & Unwin 1984
This revised edition first published in paperback by Unwin® Paperbacks,
an imprint of Unwin Hyman Limited, 1987

UNWIN HYMAN LIMITED
Denmark House, 37-39 Queen Elizabeth Street,
London SE1 2QB
and
40 Museum Street, London WC1A 1LU

Allen & Unwin Australia Pty Ltd
8 Napier Street, North Sydney, NSW 2060, Australia

Unwin Paperbacks with Port Nicholson Press
60 Cambridge Terrace, Wellington, New Zealand

British Library Cataloguing in Publication Data

Houghton, Diane
 Coping with childlessness.
1. Childlessness
I. Title   II. Houghton, Peter
362.8   HQ755.8
ISBN 0–04–649054–X

Typeset by V & M Graphics Ltd, Aylesbury, Bucks
and printed in Great Britain
by the Guernsey Press Co. Ltd,
Guernsey, Channel Islands

Contents

Acknowledgements

We should like to thank the following, all of whom greatly helped us with the book. The National Association for the Childless for access to its records; and special thanks to all those members of the Association who over the years have, by writing and talking to us, enabled us to better understand the problems of childlessness. To Brenda Holliday and her staff for their continuing help and support. To Dr Jack Glatt for his detailed comments on the medical sections. Special thanks to Maisie Smith, Linda Charlwood, the members of the National Committee, Regional Organisers and special contacts of NAC without whom this book could not have been written. To Birmingham Settlement for its support of the Association over the years and for encouraging us to write this book. To Sue Urquhart, Pauline Motzkeit, Betty Barr and Gillian Dunn for typing the manuscript, and Michael Meysel for preparing the index.

The authors wish to acknowledge that they are greatly indebted to Toni Belfield, Medical Information Officer for the Family Planning Information Service, for material incorporated in Chapter Three: 'Infertility as a medical problem', from *The Maternity Alliance Maternity Handbook* published by Penguin.

PART ONE

Infertility – the problem

1

Identifying the problem

20 December 1982

Dear Nack,

I was one of the unfortunate few who failed to resume ovulation after coming off the pill. This was in 1977 and by the end of 1978 we knew that the reason was a raised prolactin level and I was put on the drug Bromocriptine (Parlodel). This had nasty side effects but I became pregnant, only to miscarry twins at 25 weeks in November 1979. This was an all time low when we joined NAC which was a great help. I felt that I couldn't go on this awful drug again and it was two years before I tried again.

This time I took a lower dose and conceived one baby. My consultant decided to put a stitch in the neck of the womb at 15 weeks in case I had an incompetent cervix. It worked and I gave birth to a lovely baby boy on 9 December. I feel that without the help of Mr ——— at ———— Hospital I might never have had a child and am very grateful to him.

I hope that his letter will inspire anyone else on Bromocriptine who feels like giving up to give it another try. The best of luck to you all. Yours faithfully,

This letter, addressed to the quarterly newsletter of the National Association for the Childless, tells how a woman who had difficulty conceiving was helped to have a baby by the techniques of modern medicine. It is a success story, a happy resolution of a very troubling problem. There are many similar stories in the files of the National Association. They tell of babies born after extensive medical investigations, children conceived by artificial insemination, babies conceived by *in-vitro* fertilisation ('test-tube' babies), babies and older children adopted or fostered by childless couples. There are some amazing stories. They tell of the courage and persistence of individual women and men, of the care and concern of some outstanding medical practitioners, and of the hopes raised and fulfilled by modern medical science.

The staff of the Association rejoice when they receive good news of a long-awaited birth or adoption. When, however, these letters are balanced against those telling of unsuccessful attempts to become pregnant, or failed adoption applications, the unsuccessful stories seem to be more common. This would appear to be natural. It is those women in greatest need who are most likely to seek the services of the Association. Some of the letters tell of tragic lives lived out in great unhappiness. Some women's lives seem so hopeless, dogged by one disaster after another. Infertility may be compounded by redundancy, bereavement, disablement or illness. Other letters are from women whose lives were relatively tolerable until they came up against the problem of infertility. It is not only educated 'middle-class' women who write in to the Association. Women of all social classes and backgrounds pour out their experiences to a sympathetic audience.

Letters are also received from the immigrant community. The following is from an Asian woman who has great difficulty with the written language. The spelling has been corrected, but the grammar left intact where possible.

Dear Brenda,
We received your letter week before I was going for operation in ——
———————— [a private in-vitro fertilisation centre]. I had laparoscopy.
Dr ———— told me that he could not see my ovaries because of full of adhesions. He said that if I do major surgery again that could be more adhesions while we doing another laparoscopy to get the egg out. So he make me very disappointed. I think the doctor of all this reputation, he didn't help me. I am a bag of nerves nowadays.

I saw another advertisement in Childless magazine about Laser treatment in Germany for blockage of tubes and adhesions. They trying on the animals. If you got any information can you write me please.

We wanted to adopt an Asian baby as private. Please can you send us any information. We been refused by a social worker in few petty things. I am sending you a postal order for membership.
With many thanks.
P.S. We were refused for fostering, not adoption.

This woman is under pressure to have a boy child, not just to achieve a live birth. To be infertile is a great stigma for her and her husband.

The above letter describes a serious medical problem. Sometimes medical problems are compounded by other problems:

Dear Nack,
I would like to know if I have to subscribe again because I was wondering if my membership run out.

Also I have a problem which I was wondering if you could help. I wrote to you sometime back telling you that I was secondary infertile. I went to hospital and I had an internal examination. The doctor never found anything abnormal so he sent me a typed letter stating that I wasn't barren. So I told my partner. But the problem is that I am not married to my partner. But we have lived together for four years. My son is five years old now. But my partner is not his real father. But they are very close. When I told him that he is supposed to have a sperm test he didn't want to know. For the past two years he has done nothing about it. Now he has decided that he doesn't want any kids. My son is all he wants. Also when he was in his teens he had a bad pain in his scrotum. He went to hospital. But they couldn't find anything wrong. He told me that he might have a blockage. What he is frightened of is the fact that he might have a sperm test and they keep his sperms later on for a test-tube baby which he is dead against. I feel fed up of him. I nag him so much that he hardly comes home most days. I feel so depressed that I keep on crying to myself. If I did not write this down I would have felt worse.

Also I suffer from PMT and I have problems when I ovulate. The symptoms are the same. I keep getting headaches.
Thank you.
Yours faithfully,
P.S. He ripped up all of my Nack papers etc.

Though the staff of the NAC office try to send a sympathetic reply to each correspondent, a problem such as the one just described is not likely to be solved from a distance. Earlier letters from this woman also suggest that the family has financial difficulties. Where it is considered appropriate, a correspondent with a whole range of difficult problems to cope with would be referred for professional advice, if this was acceptable to them.

Letters are also received from time to time about problems experienced as a result of adoption applications. The whole topic of adoption evokes strong responses from NAC members. The insensitivity of social workers is one common theme. The inefficiency of social service departments and adoption agencies is another. Yet people are generally reluctant to pursue complaints: 'We have had a very busy, and to some extent, upsetting time. The "upsetting time" has been in connection with our British Social Services. But that is a very long chapter in itself. In fact we would write a book if we were writers.' But they are not writers. The adoption process is so painful and disturbing that it cannot be discussed, except in the greatest confidence. There must be a great fear of never receiving a child by this method, and even mentioning it to others might bring bad luck. In the same way, in times past, it was considered unlucky to display a baby's pram before a child was born. It would be tempting fate, or the devil.

How did the National Association for the Childless come into being? And what is it able to do for the childless who are faced with severe medical and social problems, such as those illustrated in the letters quoted, and many other difficulties related to problems of childlessness?

The idea for the forming of an association originated with Peter Houghton. In the course of his work as Director of a voluntary organisation involved in a variety of social and community projects, he met, from time to time, people who were suffering from a sense of pointlessness or meaninglessness. They might not have any particular social or personal problems to account for this. Indeed, many of them were comfortably off, in employment and living within a stable relationship with a partner. Sometimes they were able to be explicit about the reasons for the void in their lives. They longed for a child but they were unable to have one. People in this situation sensed a growing distance between themselves and friends of the same generation who were bringing up children, with all the energy and involvement that this entailed. Peter then undertook individual and group counselling. These childless people gained some kind of release and confidence from discussing their experiences together, and Peter wondered if perhaps their views reflected a much wider problem in society.

He advertised in the press his intentions to set up at a national level some kind of organisation for those suffering from the effects of childlessness. He did not envisage the extent of the response – 367 letters were received. Some were very sad. Here were people, not all of them young, revealing to a stranger, perhaps for the first time in their lives, their innermost distress. Some of the writers were grateful for this opportunity to communicate with a sympathetic listener, and did not ask for more. Yet many of the writers wanted the opportunity to meet with others in a similar situation, or they wanted to know where they could turn for specialist advice. The most urgent and personal letters were answered as seemed most appropriate, but there were organisational problems involved in dealing with the volume of the correspondence. Fortunately, Daphne Hughes, a social-work student on placement, was able to take over some of the secretarial work in connection with the project. Later, Elizabeth Maté introduced herself and offered to work in a voluntary capacity. Then Suzie Hayman, a member of the American National Organisation of Non-Parents and concerned with the problems of those who chose not to have children, also expressed an interest.

It was decided to hold a conference in Birmingham in March 1976. The media had been showing interest for some time, and gave publicity to the conference. There were radio interviews, television appearances and newspaper articles and, with over 80 people attending, the conference was successful. The majority were couples who had tried, unsuccessfully, to have children of their own, or to adopt. But there were also those who had chosen to remain childfree, and several representatives from adoption and social-work agencies attended, as well as researchers interested in fertility and social demography. The conference invited specialist speakers on male and female fertility, psycho-sexual problems, adoption and fostering, coming to terms with infertility, and the personal and social implications of choosing not to have children. The conference also gave an opportunity for people to meet informally, and many friendships and professional contacts were initiated.

The National Association for the Childless was formed at a General Meeting, the objectives of which were to determine policy at the national level, to focus awareness on the need for improved medical treatment of infertility, for better adoption and fostering services, and for an acceptance of the childless and valued members of society with a unique contribution to make. At a local level, the Association was to encourage the formation of self-help groups throughout the country. The local groups were to work for the improvement of services in their area, to help individual members with advice and comfort when necessary, and to arrange activities and meetings on topics of common interest.

After the Association had been in existence for a relatively short time it became clear that some kind of professional administrative structure was necessary if the Association was not to fall apart through over-rapid growth. It became a project of the Birmingham Settlement, with a paid Administrative Officer and support staff, both paid and voluntary. Liz Maté became the first Administrative Officer, and it is evident from the files how much her sensitive, caring approach was appreciated by the members. Since she left Birmingham, there have been a number of Administrative Officers, each of whom has contributed to the growth of the organisation in different ways. Rosemary Ellis helped to develop the national and regional structure of the Association, backed up by the expertise of Vanessa Constable as Information Officer. Andrew Staite added his skills as a writer and communicator. When he emigrated to Australia, the Association benfited from the extensive biological and medical knowledge of Jeremy Ward. For the last few years the administration of NAC has been in the hands of Brenda Holliday. Without her dedication and skills, the Association could not have coped with the increasing demands made upon it. Her sensitive approach has done much to comfort and reassure members going through periods of difficulty or uncertainty. She has also organised and co-ordinated a huge variety of activities, events and people, which is no mean feat with an active membership of over 4,000 at any one time, plus an even more active National Committee, Regional Committees, local groups and over one hundred local Contacts. The clerical staff and volunteers who have assisted NAC over the years have also made a vital and much-needed contribution.

The strength of the organisation lies in the co-ordination of three groups of people. There are the administrative staff in the national office, described above; there is the National Committee, led by a Chairperson, all elected annually; and there are the Regional Committees, local groups and Contacts made up from among the active membership, who work at a regional and local level.

The NAC Committee has been fortunate in being able to include in its composition both active members and professionals involved with the medical and social aspects of childlessness. Peter Houghton chaired the Committee in its first year, and was succeeded by Lindsay Carter – one of the first Committee members – who chaired the Committee for some months before she went to the Middle East. John Hilton then held the position of Chairman for several years, and his dedication and hard work were much appreciated. Barbara Mostyn, the current Chairwoman, includes among her many skills experience in the training of counsellors for self-help groups. David Owens, a sociologist from the University of Wales, Cardiff, has been in charge of NAC research since the beginning, and Lilian Llewellyn, a social worker, has advised the Association on adoption and fostering matters since 1978. The Committee's task is to formulate NAC policy at the national level, and to co-ordinate the organisation of the separate regional and local groups. It also campaigns for more effective medical treatments, brings to public awareness controversial issues such as host mothering, and presses for serious national consideration of ethical problems posed by modern scientific advances.

The work of the Regional Committees, local groups and Contacts is extremely important in the efficient running of NAC. The responsibilities of a Regional Organiser include arranging events for the regional membership, co-ordinating activities, and making doctors and fertility specialists aware of the work of NAC. In addition, local groups form in the Regions or where there is no Regional Committee offering local support. It is due to the dedication of these Regional Committees that groups are flourishing in several parts of the country. The job of a Contact is somewhat different. Contacts are generally available by telephone so that any local member in distress can discuss his or her problems with someone who has experienced the problems of infertility, for behind the concept of Regional Committees, local groups and Contacts is the belief in the value of self-help – that those who have experienced a problem are better able to advise others with a similar problem. Contacts also encourage friendship among members, and for this sensitive work they receive a training in counselling skills. Some people remain Contacts after they have had children of their own.[1]

Linking the NAC office, Committee and regional structures is the quarterly newsletter, *Issue* (formerly *NACK*) which is edited by Richard Clay. The newsletter serves a variety of purposes. It carries articles on current medical practice in infertility, and on new developments, as well as information about adoption regulations and the possibilities for adoption at home and abroad. It also provides information on current events, nationally and regionally, and has a selection of readers' letters and readers' requests. In general it is a lively magazine, much appreciated by its readers.

What has been achieved by NAC since its inception in 1976? In the area of medical treatments it has undoubtedly had some success, particularly in attracting some of the most outstanding fertility specialists to give of their time and talents to the Association. It has also promoted an awareness of the needs of the infertile at a national level. Compared with what was available only a few years ago, several small miracles have occurred through advances in the understanding and treatment of female infertility. The most spectacular has been the 'test-tube baby', but a variety of other treatments have also brought hope to many women. Male fertility is also better understood, although there have not been any advances as spectacular as those for women. The nature of infertility as a joint problem between male and female in a relationship is also better understood.

Surveying the national provision for fertility treatments, it is evident that some areas are better served than others, and that it is still necessary for many couples to seek treatment privately, because of the low priority accorded to fertility treatments within the National Health Service. As a result, NAC is at present considering whether to set up its own fertility clinic. The NAC office contains a variety of articles on the medical aspects of infertility which are available to members, and it can call on the services of medical specialists for advice on particular problems. The drug company, Serono Ltd, has very kindly helped with the organisation and sponsorship of a series of symposia throughout the country on the medical aspects of infertility.

Concerning adoption, NAC has developed contacts with a number of societies, and also provides its membership with advice and assistance. The main problem has been that each year there are fewer babies or young children available for adoption, and this traditional avenue to children for the childless has virtually closed. Several adoption societies and social service departments have in recent years become much more sensitive to the feelings of the childless who are going through assessment procedures, but it is likely that many couples who would in the past have applied to adopt are now seeking treatment by artificial insemination. Thus, the importance of medical treatments is increasing, as there are so few social solutions. Inter-country adoptions have been explored, but UK law on adoption has become stricter, and bureaucratic procedures in other countries are usually cumbersome. Among NAC members it is the older childless who tend to seek inter-country adoption, probably because this represents their only hope for a child.

The most difficult yet challenging aspect of NAC's work lies in helping members who are denied children to come to terms with their situation, and to develop a new approach to life that is based on an alternative to children. Relatively little is known about the common features of successful adaption, and this book is one attempt to remedy this. However, judging from the NAC files, it is evident that large numbers of members use the Association to help them to achieve a child at almost any cost. It was originally envisaged that the involuntary childless and those who had chosen not to have children would work together to encourage a greater awareness of the social value of life without children, but this did not happen. The two groups had very little in common. They opposed each other in meetings and each side accused the other of being 'selfish'. (This made us think that the word served no useful purpose and should be banned from the language.) Suzie Hayman eventually set up a separate organisation for those who chose life without children. This separation is regretted, as each side does have something positive to learn from the other.

In NAC much valuable work is done by local Contacts in helping the childless to reconcile themselves to their situation, and to begin to think positively about alternatives. Contacts, as part of their training, are taught to listen sensitively, and to suggest the possibility of an alternative perspective where appropriate. Members of the National Committee are sometimes called upon to offer advice, and Peter Houghton deals with adjustment problems by telephone or in private interviews. Adjustment is a very long-term process, and often a successful outcome can only be determined negatively, in that the member has left the Association because he or she no longer has a need for its services. It is difficult to quantify results in this important area of NAC's work, as so much of it is confidential. It is also very difficult to lay down general rules as to what constitutes successful adjustment.

There is not much written about coming to terms with childlessness. There are some excellent books on the medical aspects of infertility, many of which contain a chapter on alternatives.[2] But there is an absence of detailed treatment on the subject. Statistics on infertility[3] would suggest that large numbers of people have to accept that they will not have children of their own, and most of these do find some way of coping with life. The majority are not seen as a group needing special help. Many would find it hard to describe how they came to terms with their situation and, for some, it may not even be an issue of concern. Nevertheless, there is sufficient evidence within the Association and elsewhere to suggest that there *is* a current need for help and advice in coping with childlessness.

This book aims to provide some of the needed help and advice for those who are faced with the prospect of a life without their own children. It may also, it is hoped, provide a means to greater understanding of the problems of childlessness among the general public, and among those professionals who deal with the involuntary childless.

2

Who are the childless?

A person who has not borne or fathered a child is childless in the broad definition of this word. This is not, however, what is generally meant when 'childless couples' or 'the childless' are referred to. The term 'childless', if it is to be of use in any discussion of difficulties or problems experienced by 'the childless', has to be given a more specific meaning. At the same time this meaning has to include an emotional component, if 'childlessness' is to be fully understood.

In attempting to define 'childless', it is probably easier to decide first those categories of people who are *not* included in the more specific meaning of the term. Children and adolescents are not included. Pre-adolescents are not biologically equipped to become mothers or fathers. And the period of early adolescence is generally regarded as an inappropriate stage of life for young people to become parents. This is certainly the case in the West. In other parts of the world it might be possible to consider a young adolescent married woman who had not borne a child to be 'childless'. The term would not, however, be applied to her husband, even if he had good grounds for considering himself to be medically infertile.

There are several major social groups who, because of the nature of their life-style, are not considered to be childless in the sense under discussion at this point. Single people without children are assumed to be childless only in the very general sense of the word. Though some single people have children, and raise them themselves, being single does not of itself imply childlessness. Many single people do, however, regret and mourn their childless status in similar ways to those who are married or in a long-term relationship with a partner. In terms of how they feel, many, but not all, single people are childless in outlook. The difference between the single and others is that the single are much less likely to be undergoing treatment for infertility. Many single people may never have cause to discover whether they are fertile or infertile in medical terms.

Another group excluded from the more specific meaning of 'childless' are those who make a deliberate choice not to have children. It is likely that many of these people will practice some form of birth control during their fertile years. A woman may wish to pursue a demanding career, or feel that her contribution to society could be more effective if she was without the restrictions imposed on her by motherhood. A man may find that the idea of fatherhood conflicts with his most important aims in life. There are many examples of this. Catholic nuns and priests give up their right to have children and their right to a sexual relationship for what they see as the greater cause of service to God and human-kind. Many people consider themselves to be 'childfree' by choice, emphasising the positive nature of their decision, and stressing for themselves the negative implications of parenthood.[1]

As contraception, abortion and sterilisation have become more widely accepted as means to birth control and family planning, women have been given greater freedom to choose the future direction of their lives, and the numbers seeking to avoid parenthood have grown. In earlier generations the only way to do this was to remain unmarried, thus denying oneself a heterosexual physical relationship for life, or until the woman's childbearing years were over. There was, therefore, a population of single women to be found in many service professions such as teaching, nursing and domestic service. Nowadays no one need necessarily forego sexuality as well as parenthood. Those women who are absolutely determined against having children may, at some point during their fertile years, have a sterilization, and men sometimes decide to have a vasectomy, although probably more often to limit the size of a family, rather than to ensure that there will be no children at all.

There have always been people who did not wish to parent, but this is the first generation where people can choose not to have children without paying too high a price in personal and social terms. The intention not to parent no longer requires prolonged single status, with all that this implies in terms of loneliness and sexual self-discipline. It has meant, too, that marriage is no longer necessary as a prelude to a long-standing sexual partnership, and pregnancy is no longer the inevitable result of a sexual relationship. Marriage now survives primarily because of the need for commitment and partnership, though many may still feel that it exists to protect the children of a union during their formative years. The large numbers of divorces where children are involved would, however, suggest that marriage as an institution for the benefit of children takes second place when the relationship between the parents is at issue. 'Staying together for the sake of the children' is no longer accepted as a universally valid solution to a marital problem. Thus, with the wider availability of family planning techniques has come a greater questioning of the purpose of marriage, and a greater awareness of the importance of the decision as to whether or not one should have children.

In considering the question 'Who are the childless?' it has been necessary to think about the childfree, because the distinction between them and the childless can become rather confused. Both feel similarly the social pressure from peers, parents, relatives and society in general to bear children. The fundamental difference may be obscured, however, by their common problems. The objective of one group is to have children. The objective of the other is not to have children. Because of this major difference in intention, the childfree are not considered to be 'childless' in the special sense required for the purposes of the present discussion.

There are a number of minority groups who are commonly without children. Homosexuals and lesbians are usually childless unless they have chosen their preferred sexual role after a heterosexual partnership which has produced children. For lesbian women today there is a possibility of having a child by artificial insemination of donated sperm, and this does mean that the choice of or preference for lesbian sexuality no longer implies a consequent choice of childlessness. Such is not the case for homosexual men, for whom childlessness, however much regretted, is inevitable.

The bereaved are another social group. Some will be people whose partners died early within a relationship, before marriage, or before the woman was able to conceive. The partner's death may have been through tragic circumstances, and the surviving partner has not entered into any other lasting relationship. The bereaved will also include those who are made childless because of miscarriage, stillbirth or the death of a child during the parents' lifetime.

There has been a change in the type of person constituting the first category of the bereaved. In the first half of this century the effect of two world wars was to reduce the male population, leaving many widows childless. There was also a greater likelihood of a person dying at a young age from one of several major diseases for which there was then no known cure. The female partners of men who died young did not have a chance to receive artificial insemination by donor to give them the opportunity to become a single parent after their bereavement. Nowadays, because of the widespread use of contraception, some young women may be deprived of children through their partner's death, where half a century ago they would most likely have produced at least one child fairly soon after marriage, in the absence of effective contraception. A child, in such circumstances, comes to have a symbolic meaning. A woman may wish she had borne a child so that 'something of my husband remains'. A woman who had been able to give birth said 'My little girl is all that my husband achieved in his life'.

Another group for whom childlessness may become an unintended consequence is where there is a large gap in age between a couple.

Fertility generally decreases with age, for both sexes, although the man's decline is usually more prolonged than the woman's, and such couples may have problems when the woman tries to conceive. The older partner may fear being replaced by someone younger and more fertile, and can become jealous. The younger partner may fear early bereavement and experience a failing sexual responsiveness from the other partner. The intensity of the desire for a child may be greater in one partner than the other, leading to increased stress within the relationship. It may not always be the younger partner who has the greater need to parent, and as time passes the desire of the older partner for a child may become overwhelming.

Adoptive or foster parents may also be childless in a physical sense, even though they are bringing up their 'own' children. For many people, adoption brings to an end the feeling of being childless, but not in all cases. Some adoptive parents differ among themselves in the intensity of their desire for a child, and one aspect of a social worker's assessment of prospective adopters is to discover the extent to which both partners are in agreement on this issue. There are cases of later rejection of the adopted children by one partner for a variety of reasons. It is a little ironic that adoption is often seen as the obvious solution for the childless, when it is not always preferred. The advent of donor insemination has given rise to disquiet on the part of many infertile male partners, but research suggests that AID seems preferred to adoption because 'at least one partner has a child of their own'.[2]

There is, finally, a category of people whom it would be difficult to describe as childless, in that they or their partner have given birth to a surviving child. But the intensity of the desire for another child is increased when there are problems leading to the woman's failure to conceive or carry a subsequent pregnancy to full term. This is usually called 'secondary infertility'. Sometimes there are medical reasons for this, but these may be complicated by social problems. One partner may have had a sterilization or vasectomy which has proved irreversible. Sometimes a partner re-marries, and wishes to establish a second family. Where both partners have been married before, and completed their families, there may still be a need for them to have a child, as they wish to strengthen their new relationship. Their strong desire to have a child may meet with total incomprehension.

When I told the gynaecologist how we so desperately wanted a child of our own, he just laughed in my face and said it was out of the question. We talked to another GP who says we must make the best of the children we have and are lucky to have them. What doctors can't understand is the children are not *ours*. If only we could have the operations reversed it would change our lives.

Such a couple as this would appear to belong to the category of the childless, even though between them they have been responsible for the births of five children.

How, then, can one define a category of people suffering from the effects of childlessness, that on the one hand excludes those who have good reasons for not wanting to be included in the category, but on the other enables the inclusion of the various groups shown to be childless in the ways described above. It would seem that inability to have one's own biological child at some point has to be part of the definition. There also needs to be room in the definition to incorporate the emotional impact of failing to have a child. In some of the categories of the childless discussed, infertility is not necessarily a factor and the medical term 'infertility' is evidently not an adequate definition for these purposes. Just as, conversely, already having one's own children is not a necessary disqualification from feeling childless.

If one starts, however, with the simplest case, that of a young or youngish couple wanting to start a family but experiencing difficulties in achieving this, one could list the following essential components in a definition of childlessness:

1. children are desired, but medical problems or social circumstances lead to difficulties in having children.
2. the absence of children leads to a sense of being deprived or thwarted, and there is a feeling of grief or loss.
3. ways to have children are actively sought.

This definition would include a majority of those who contact the National Association for the Childless for help or advice. But it still leaves out a sizeable number of people who would consider themselves childless.

The most obvious category omitted is that of people who are past child-bearing age. Additionally, there are those who for a variety of reasons are not actively seeking children, though they may have taken steps to achieve them at some earlier time. There may also be some who have been unsuccessful in having a family, who once grieved, but now are reconciled to their condition. The following slightly broader definition would seem to incorporate the categories not covered in the first definition:

4. parenting is or was regarded as an important aim in life.
5. grief and loss are or were experienced when difficulty in achieving this aim is or was encountered.
6. despite some resolution of the problem, the feeling of loss or regret persists, though not necessarily at all times or with the same amount of intensity.

The emphasis with this second definition is on the emotional impact of childlessness upon the lives of those who experience it. The medical conception of the state of infertility is not excluded from this second definition, but it is very much subordinated to the emotional aspect of the problems of childlessness. Both definitions serve useful purposes. The first one is a good working definition for those involved with the younger childless in a professional capacity. It suggests that a full understanding of childlessness during the 'fertile' years needs to include an understanding of the whole personality, and if gynaecologists and social workers, among others, can appreciate the special needs of the childless, that is all to the good. However, for the purposes of this book the second definition is likely to prove more relevant, in that, particularly in Part Two, the emphasis is on the emotional impact of childlessness as it extends throughout and beyond the period usually characterised as the childbearing years.

When one tries to assess the size of the problem of childlessness it is difficult to obtain accurate statistics. As has been suggested above there is a distinction between those for whom childlessness is a problem, and those for whom it is not. Among those affected by childlessness, a distinction needs to be made between those young enough to benefit from available solutions to the problem, and those who are past an age where childbirth of child-rearing can reasonably be expected of them.

The available statistics suggest that about 15 per cent of the UK adult population of childbearing age is childless (primarily infertile) in the broad sense, i.e. that they have not had a surviving child up to the present time.[3] A survey by Andrew Stanway of the quoted statistics gives rates between 11 and 22 per cent.[4] Looking at the available statistics another way, John Stangel suggested in 1979 that the pregnancy rates of sexually active women of childbearing age provide a useful way to assess the likely extent of fertility problems among the population as a whole. He estimated the length of time required for a normally fertile woman (having unprotected sex) to become pregnant. His figures are.[5]

after one month of sexual relations – 25 per cent will be pregnant.
after six months – 63 per cent
after nine months – 75 per cent
after twelve months – 80 per cent
after eighteen months – 90 per cent

These figures are not broken down by age, which is an important omission, as the peak period of female fertility occurs in the mid-twenties or earlier. We can assume that the older the woman, the more likely it is that she will take longer to conceive. Stangel's figures suggest that anyone not pregnant after eighteen months of trying for a baby should seek medical help. If one takes the age factor into account it would be advisable to consider asking for help after six months.

However, the most valuable piece of research into the likely incidence of infertility in a population has been carried out by Michael Hull and his colleagues in the Bristol area. His findings would seem reasonably representative of the situation in other parts of the country. They looked at 708 couples who attended a clinic for the first time in one particular year; most attended one particular clinic. The couples had all been infertile for at least one year, and the average period was two and a half years.

The annual incidence represented 1.2 couples per thousand total population. The lifetime incidence was 17% – that is, about one in six couples appeared to need the help of a specialist infertility clinic at some time in their lives. One in eight needed help for a first child, and many couples would fail to have a child.[6]

It is possible to measure the numbers of people who are defined as childless under our first definition (p. 16), but there is no way of measuring the extent of the distress caused by childlessness in our second sense. Elliot Philipp does attempt to include the emotional impact of childlessness within the scope of his estimates: 'There are at least one million couples in the United Kingdom who are at this moment wishing for a baby or a pregnancy, and have been trying for years to achieve their desire.[7]

In a later book, commenting on the organisation of a particular fertility team, he suggests that although very few of his patients require psychiatric help, the remaining 95 per cent do require psychological support.[8] Thus, both his estimates of the extent of the problem nationally, and his figures for his own clinic, support the suggestions implicit in many of the other statistics, that childlessness as a problem is of some considerable size, and that it may even be on the increase.

Barbara Eck Menning, writing in 1977 about the situation in the United States, and Andrew Stanway writing about the UK both suggest that infertility is becoming more common.[9] The reasons they give are of some importance for an understanding of how changes in social attitudes and behaviour can lead to changes in birth rates. The first, and most prominent, reason is that couples are choosing to delay marriage and childbirth (particularly the latter) into their late twenties and early thirties, when women are less fertile. Thus, many more couples may need medical help if the woman is to conceive, and some couples may not be able to conceive at all. Another reason given is the rise in the incidence of venereal disease, particularly among teenagers. About 18 per cent of women suffering from gonorrhoea will have inflammation of the fallopian tubes, thus preventing fertilisation of the egg. Birth-control methods also cause problems for a small percentage of those who use the contraceptive pill or an intra-uterine device. The figures for this are small in relation to the number of users. Of roughly 3½ million women using the pill, about 70,000 will be affected (about 2 per cent). These 70,000 will form about 8 per cent of the one million estimated to need help in becoming pregnant. A fourth cause is thought to be exposure to drugs, environmental pollution, restricting clothes such as tight male underwear, and nutritional deficiencies.

The fall in levels of fertility poses social and economic problems for the developed countries, where some populations are reaching zero growth, and others are falling. East and West Germany, Austria and Luxembourg all appear to have falling populations. The UK, USSR, USA, France and the Scandinavian countries are slowly reaching that point.[10] This will, over the next few decades, lead to changes in the distribution of the different age groups within those populations. With an increasing burden of frail elderly, each of these countries will be faced with the need to make policy decisions about the most effective ways to redress the balance, in order to ensure that there will be a younger population of sufficient size and productive power to support and maintain the older generations in reasonably humane conditions. The future of the childless in the developed world will be very much affected by national policy decisions on population matters. It remains to be seen whether individual countries will regard the childless as a potentially valuable resource, and encourage the development of new fertility treatments. Or will there be a continuation of the present indecision that prevails in many of these countries, leaving the childless socially in a kind of no-man's land, and psychologically in a state of continuing distress?

3

Infertility as a medical problem

Though the emphasis of the present book is upon childlessness as a problem which affects the emotions and reactions of those who are unable to have children, it has to be remembered that *infertility* is primarily a *medical* problem. One reason for our decision not to emphasise the medical aspects of childlessness was that there are several good descriptions of the problems of infertility already available.[1] For those readers most interested in the biological and medical accounts of fertility, most of the books recommended in the reading list on pages 170–2 cover the area in much greater detail than is done in this chapter. Our purpose here is to *outline* the major factors determining whether a woman becomes pregnant, the possible causes of difficulty in conceiving, and the treatments available to a couple who wish to start their own family and who need medical help to achieve this. This medical description will act as a background to later chapters which will attempt to show that inability to have a child of one's own has consequences which are at the same time *physical*, *social* and *emotional*.

How a woman becomes pregnant

Each month a fertile woman releases an egg from one of her ovaries. The egg must travel from the ovary through the fallopian tubes into the womb. In the fallopian tubes it has to encounter sperm from the man, and the sperm has to penetrate and fertilise the egg. The egg lives only a short time and thus it has to be fertilised near to ovulation (this is about 14 days *before* the next due period). The sperm is deposited during intercourse in the vagina near its entrance (the cervix). Intercourse needs to take place near the time of ovulation, as sperm only live for a short time. The sperm swim up through the womb to meet the egg in the fallopian tubes. Many die on the way, so sperm have both to be able to swim and to exist in sufficient quantity to make it possible that at least one of the sperm might reach the egg. The fertilised egg moves down into the womb (uterus) and implants itself in the womb lining, where the embryo can develop.

To summarise, a woman must release an egg in mid-menstrual cycle; this egg must be able to both enter and to travel down the fallopian tubes. The man's sperm must be able to reach the egg through the woman's upper vagina, cervix and womb, and the lower ends of the fallopian tubes. The sperm must be able to penetrate the egg, and the fertilised egg must then move down into the womb, and become implanted in the womb lining.

There are several factors complicating the reproductive cycle described above. Age is one factor. A woman who is in her thirties will not conceive as quickly as a woman in her twenties, so younger women who want a family later than is usual need to take account of the fact they may have more difficulty conceiving when they are older. Alcohol abuse may affect the number and viability of the sperm produced by men. Intercourse needs to take place as close to ovulation as possible, and good penetration of the vagina lessens the distance the ejaculated sperm has to travel and ensures the sperm is placed as advantageously as possible for the journey. Problems in successfully completing sexual intercourse, or the use of a position during intercourse that does not allow the man's penis to penetrate high enough up the woman's vagina, can adversely affect the ability of sperm to penetrate the woman's cervix and womb, and to move onwards into the fallopian tubes.

It is possible for a woman to ascertain whether she is ovulating or not by taking her basal body temperature first thing in the morning before rising. If ovulation takes place, the basal body temperature will rise, around the middle of the monthly cycle, by up to half a degree centigrade, and will remain at that level until the next period begins (end of the cycle). If intercourse is timed to roughly coincide with the rise in temperature it can help conception, since at no other time is the egg in the fallopian tubes or is the sperm able to penetrate the cervix. The cervix is lined with mucus-secreting glands. During ovulation, as the result of the release of the hormones oestrogen and progesterone from the ovary, the mucus alters, becoming less thick and sticky, and more watery, thus removing a crucial barrier to the sperm. Woman are often advised to stay still for about half an hour after having intercourse at such times, to enable the cervix to be bathed in sperm.

Fertility investigations

The investigation and treatment of infertility is usually undertaken via the National Health Service, although it is also available privately. An individual or couple worried about a possible fertility problem almost always consult their NHS general practitioner as a first step. If the GP feels that the couple have not been practising intercourse with a view to conception for very long, he or she may sometimes suggest that the couple should persevere for a few more months, and the woman patient may be given advice about the importance of keeping a temperature chart. More often, however, a GP will refer the woman patient, or the couple, to a hospital that is known to undertake infertility investigations. The GP is not an expert in the field of infertility, and he or she must refer a patient for specialist help.

The first visit to a clinic is important. It is during the first consultation that a medical history is taken, and questions will be asked about a couple's patterns of sexual intercourse, to ascertain if a sexual or emotional problem has arisen. Most clinics try to see both partners at the beginning of an investigation, although there are still some men who refuse to accompany their partner to the clinic. Usually there is an opportunity for the patient to discuss the type of investigation and treatment being offered, and how they are likely to be suitable in the individual case. It is important that, wherever possible, both partners are included in this initial discussion.

Most clinics in hospitals that undertake infertility investigations are based within the gynaecological service. This means that only where a gynaecologist has a special interest in the subject will a full range of services be easily available. There are some hospitals which have an infertility clinic that specialises in the diagnosis and treatment of infertility problems, and these centres of excellence are much in demand, as the best and more advanced treatment is usually only available in such places. Infertility, if it is to be properly treated, cannot be regarded as simply a gynaecological problem. A patient may need to see other specialists such as endocrinologists, andrologists and immunologists. Most gynaecology clinics are, however, able to carry out basic tests. If these tests indicate that a patient may need treatment or further investigations which are not readily available in the gynaecology clinic, it is suggested that he or she should ask if they can be referred to the nearest centre that specialises in the investigation and treatment of infertility. This request should be made tactfully, as consultants may resent the implied criticisms of their own services.

It can be distressing to infertility patients if they find that the gynaecologist does not separate fertility cases from his or her other patients. An infertile woman may be treated alongside expectant mothers, women with post-natal problems, and women undergoing hysterectomies or abortions. However, most hospitals now try to ensure minimum contact among these different kinds of patient. Where there is still a policy of mixing them, it would indicate that a low priority is given to infertility treatment, or that the hospital authorities are insensitive to the needs of the different types of patients.

Investigations and treatment may take a considerable time, depending upon where a couple are sent, whom they see, and upon the nature of any fertility problem subsequently discovered. Waiting lists may be long in some areas, so that a period of time may elapse even before investigations are begun. There is often a long gap between subsequent appointments, and sometimes a patient may see a different doctor each time. Some of these doctors may be unfamiliar with particular cases. The time allowed to elapse between appointments, and the lack of continuity in medical personnel are major complaints made by infertility patients. Both lead the patient to believe that his or her case has a low priority, and that the hospital or department is not really interested in infertility problems. Sometimes it may seem that a solution will never be found, and that treatment may be carried on for years. Some clinics do, however, manage to arrange treatments so that delay is minimised, the patient sees at least one member of the hospital staff on a continuous basis, and the patient receives a clear explanation of what is happening, and why, at each stage of treatment. It is the practice of the very few good clinics that highlights the poverty of the response to infertility problems in the many inadequate or indifferent departments.

There is, however, another reason why an investigation may sometimes take a considerable time to complete. Primarily, this is because so many of the tests have to be performed around the timing of the woman's menstrual cycle; ovulation only takes place once a month. Another reason for a possible delay is that the results of some treatments may take time to assess. Hormone drugs do not usually have an immediate effect, and may need to be taken for a prescribed length of time before they are likely to affect ovulation. A woman who undergoes micro-surgery to unblock her fallopian tubes will need an extended period of time to assess the success of the operation, as this may occur within a year or two or as easily as within a few months. The nature of the problem, and the complications of the relevant treatment, may mean, therefore, that some patients may find themselves undergoing treatment or investigations for several years.

While clinics vary as to the type of tests they undertake, and the order in which these tests are carried out, the main investigations and treatments tend to be carried out in the same order. The investigation of the man's fertility is begun, where possible, at the same time that the woman's fertility is being investigated.

Common female infertility problems

The problems experienced by women are mainly of two kinds. Firstly, they may have a problem with ovulation – they may fail to ovulate, or may have a hormonal imbalance or deficiency affecting the efficiency of their ovulation. Women with this problem may be unable to release eggs from their ovaries in the normal way, or they may be releasing eggs into their fallopian tubes with insufficient regularity. Secondly, women may have a mechanical blockage, or some deformity in their reproductive system that prevents their egg from reaching the man's sperm, or vice-versa. These two important problems of female infertility will now be discussed separately, though it should be remembered that they may be interrelated in some individual cases.

(a) OVULATORY PROBLEMS

1. *Failure to ovulate*
Nearly all women of child-bearing age who are functioning normally ovulate approximately once a month. This happens because certain hormonal changes take place during the monthly cycle. Two main hormones control these changes – oestrogen and progesterone. There may be a variety of reasons for ovulatory failure, and it is possible to investigate the causes by means of a variety of tests. Once a test or series of tests has revealed a woman's inability to ovulate naturally, there is a choice of treatments available for the possible solution of an individual ovulation problem.

Possible causes

(i)   The gonadotrophic hormones produced by the pituitary gland (which is situated near the brain) may fail to stimulate the ripening of an egg within the ovary; or else the hormones may fail to stimulate the release of the ripened egg into the fallopian tubes. Two hormones are involved. FSH (follicle stimulating hormone) triggers the ripening of the egg and the production of oestrogen. LH (luteinising hormone) stimulates the release of the egg and the production of progesterone.

(ii)   There may be a reduced number of eggs in the ovary (a woman usually has about 100,000 eggs, stored from birth).

(iii)   There may have been damage to the ovaries, often as a result of exposure to previous surgery, endometriosis or inflammation.

(iv)   There may be hormonal disorders, such as a raised prolactin level (prolactin is a hormone which triggers the production of milk in the breasts). Another hormonal problem is the malfunction of the thyroid (this is a gland which produces a hormone, thyroxine, which is involved in the release of energy from the body tissues).

Investigation

(i) The basal body temperature (BBT) is monitored. This involves the woman taking her temperature after rest and *before* any activity. As there is a small temperature change when an egg is released, the temperature chart shows whether ovulation is occurring. This can be difficult to chart if ovulation is irregular, as the length of a monthly cycle will vary.

(ii) The cervical mucus is observed around the time of ovulation, as the mucus then should become less thick and sticky, making it more easily penetrated by sperm. A thick, sticky mucus suggests that the levels of oestrogen secreted are inadequate and that ovulation may not have occurred.

(iii) Blood and urine tests can be made to find out what hormones are present. This test can also indicate whether ovulation has occurred.

(iv) More recently, ultrasound scanners have been used. These scanners can display the ovaries on a screen, and can show if the egg has been released, or is in process of being released.

(v) An endometrial biopsy (removal of a small portion of the lining of the womb) can also be taken in the second half of the monthly cycle. This is to show whether progesterone has been released, as would be the case if ovulation had occurred.

Treatment If the above tests reveal that there is a problem with ovulation, there are several treatments available. Their purpose is to stimulate the process of ovulation.

(i) Fertility drugs. These are given over a period of time. Clomiphene, a synthetic compound, may be taken orally. If the gonadotrophins, containing FSH and LH, are used, these are given by injection under clinic supervision. The two types used in this way are human menopausal gonadotrophin and human chorionic gonadotrophin.

(ii) Hormone pump. This can be attached to the arm, and used to inject tiny quantities of FSH and LH releasing hormone via a needle inserted under the skin. The releasing hormone then directly stimulates the pituitary gland to produce its own FSH and LH.

(iii) Bromocriptine. This drug has a variety of uses, including the control of Parkinson's disease. It is also used to reduce abnormally high prolactin levels in women, as this causes ovulation problems.

2. *Hormonal imbalance or deficiency*

Here the oestrogen, progesterone and other necessary hormones are produced within a woman's body, but are not fulfilling their normal function. Ovulation may be prevented, or the pattern of the cycle may be changed. The cervical mucus may not be thinned in time, the egg may be prevented from being implanted in the lining of the womb, or a pregnancy may not be able to proceed to full term because of lack of suitable conditions for the fertilised egg (embryo) within the womb. The main effect of a hormonal imbalance or deficiency is to prevent penetration of the woman's egg by male sperm.

Possible causes

(i)   Too low levels of oestrogen and progesterone.
(ii) diabetes; or thyroid, adrenal or prolactin disorders.

Investigation   A post-coital test may be needed to see whether sperm is moving, or has moved, through the woman's cervical mucus, a few hours after intercourse has taken place. If there are difficulties here, the sperm may be unable to reach the egg, or to fertilise it. The test involves the examination of samples of vaginal and cervical secretions.

Treatment   The main treatment for this condition is to ensure ovulation by giving ovulation-inducing drugs where necessary. Mid-cycle oestrogens may be given when a poor post-coital test is due to unusually thick or scanty mucus.

3. *Blockage or abnormality in the reproductive organs*

A blockage or abnormality of the reproductive organs prevents fertilisation of the egg, by closing the pathway between the egg and the sperm. Such a problem may also prevent the implantation of the fertilised egg in the womb lining. If there is a problem inside the womb, a pregnancy may be unable to develop.

Possible causes

(i)   Scar tissue or adhesions. Here, fibrous tissues may block or hold together the sides of the fallopian tubes, thus preventing the egg from moving through them. These scar tissues or adhesions can occur as a result of an abdominal operation or a pelvic infection.

(ii) Endometriosis. Endometrial tissues can block off both tubes, cause adhesions, or damage the ovaries. These tissues are small pieces of the womb lining, which is usually evacuated at the end of the cycle. The tissues have, for some reason, implanted themselves outside the womb, and have grown in size.

(iii) Fibroids, polyps. These are benign tissue growths within the womb that can become large enough to cause blockage, or prevent an embryo from implanting.

(iv) Abnormally-shaped womb or fallopian tubes; the womb or tubes may also be malformed.

(v) Weak cervix. This is where the cervix is not strong enough to hold a baby in, as it grows within the womb.

Investigation   It is normal, if a blockage or abnormality of the reproductive organs is suspected, to give the patient a general physical examination. This is to see if there are any apparent reasons to expect a blockage or abnormality. Three main tests may then be used to continue the investigation, although the first (the laparoscopy) is increasingly replacing the other two.

(i) A laparoscopic investigation involves a small operation during which a small telescope-like instrument (a laparoscope) is introduced into the internal abdominal organs, through a tiny incision in the abdomen. This enables the reproductive organs to be viewed directly. In some cases samples of the fluids in the organs can also be taken, to test for hormone levels and the presence of sperm etc. The operation is usually done under a general anaesthetic.

(ii) A hysterosalpinogram may also be used. Here a radio-opaque dye is injected through the vagina into the reproductive organs. An X-ray is then taken, so that the inside of the organs can be seen and the problem area identified.

(iii) An air insufflation test (Rubin's Test) is sometimes carried out, though rarely nowadays, as it is rather unreliable and has largely been supplanted by the hysterosalpinogram and laparoscopy. In the air insufflation test, carbon dioxide is blown into the womb under pressure. The level of the pressure is observed, and if the tubes are not blocked the gas escapes harmlessly, and pressure will be felt by the woman in the area of her shoulder.

Treatment   There has been less success with treatment for this kind of problem than there has been with ovulation problems. The main treatments are:

(i)   Microsurgery within the fallopian tubes to remove a blockage.

(ii)   Surgery to correct any abnormality, for example, the removal of adhesions (fibroids, polyps, endometrial tissues). This may have only limited success, because the adhesions may be widespread and cannot all be removed, or because they may recur.

(iii)   A special stitch (the Shirodkar stitch). This is made in order to strengthen a weak cervix during pregnancy, and is removed before labour.

(iv)   *In-vitro* fertilisation. This has recently become available in a few specialised centres. It involves the fertilisation of the woman's egg outside the body in laboratory conditions. An egg, mature and ready for fertilisation, is removed from the ovary by laparoscopy, and put in a special fluid in a laboratory glass container.The sperm of the male partner is then added. If fertilisation is observed to have taken place, and the embryo subsequently begins to develop, the embryo is then placed in the mother's womb. The hope is that the embryo will be able to plant itself in the lining of the womb in the normal way.

Male infertility problems

A fertile man normally produces sperm in both his testes (testicles). It takes about ten to twelve weeks to complete a set of sperm potentially capable of travelling through a woman's vagina, cervix and womb, and to fertilise an egg in one of her fallopian tubes. Anything that interferes with the production of sperm within the testes has an effect on the quantity or quality of sperm, or both. The two main infertility problems of men are, firstly, low sperm production (oligo-spermia) or failure to produce any sperm (azoospermia); secondly, sperm may not be of the right size and shape, and may not be able to move (swim) freely after ejaculation (impaired motility).

Possible causes   Production and motility (potential for movement) are affected by a variety of factors:

(i)   Inadequate production of the gonadotrophic hormones FSH and LH. As in the woman's reproductive system, the male system is dependent on the release of FSH and LH from the pituitary gland. These two hormones are necessary for the production of testosterone, the hormone that is necessary for the development of 'maleness' in a man, and is also required for the efficient production of healthy sperm, and seminal fluid (the liquid in which the sperm are contained at the point of ejaculation into the woman's vagina).

(ii) Certain illnesses that can cause tissue damage in the testes. Normal sperm development is thereby prevented. Mumps is one example of an illness that can, in some cases, prevent sperm development.

(iii) Blockage of the vas deferens tubes. These tubes normally carry sperm from the man's testes to his penis, but they may become blocked for some reason.

(iv) Undescended testicles (cryptorchidism). Here the testes have remained within the abdomen, rather than dropping into the scrotum at birth. The testes do not grow properly, and sperm is not developed within the testes.

(v) Smoking, drugs, alcohol and too high a temperature of the testes. All of these can affect the normal production and development of sperm. Men are sometimes advised to avoid tight underwear during fertility treatment, in order to keep the testes from becoming overheated.

(vi) Immune problems. For reasons which are as yet unclear, the man's body or the woman's cervical mucus may produce antibodies which attack the sperm, and thus kill the sperm or prevent their passage to the egg. Sometimes the effect of antibodies is to clump the sperm together, and prevent their free movement.

(vii) Ejaculation problems. These may occur when a man's penis is unable to become sufficiently rigid for it to enter the woman's vagina. This may be the result of a physical disability, or a problem with sexual intercourse. Drugs used to treat hypertension are also thought to cause ejaculation problems if used regularly over a long period.

(viii) Varicoceles. These are varicose veins around the testis which can develop in some men and may impair sperm numbers or motility. This occurs due to increased local heat or toxins produced by these swollen veins.

(ix) Unknown causes. Unfortunately this is the commonest category.

Investigation Various fairly simple investigations are possible to establish whether any of the above factors are present:

(i) A specimen of semen is usually obtained first. The man is asked to ejaculate by masturbation, and the ejaculate is collected in a container. The sperm are then examined to check whether there are enough of them to make fertilisation likely, and whether the sperm are of sufficiently good quality to perform the tasks required of them (they must be of the right shape, size and motility). It is usually necessary to take at least two samples of sperm on different occasions. Sperm are laid down in the testes about ten weeks prior to any ejaculation; and environment, health and other factors can affect their quality and numbers.

(ii)   The post coital test carried out on the woman (see page 27) can also be used to check that the man is able to place his sperm into the womb successfully.

(iii) A testicular biopsy can also be carried out, usually under a general anaesthetic. Tissues from each of the testes are removed for examination. The aim is to assess whether sperm production is possible, and whether it is actually taking place within the testes.

(iv)   A vasography is used to check whether the vas deferens are free from blockage, and is usually done at the same time as a testicular biopsy. Vasography is an X-ray technique which uses radio-opaque dye to show up any blockage.

Treatment   Male infertility is difficult to treat. Though there are several treatments in use, the results are not generally very satisfactory.

(i)   Surgery can be used to unblock the vas deferens or remove varicose veins.

(ii)   Fertility drugs such as clomiphene and testosterone may be used, to try to boost sperm production and improve sperm quality.

(iii) Steroids may be used to try to combat the formation of antibodies.

(iv)   Advice may be given about the importance of wearing looser clothing, or bathing the testes in cool water. Alcohol and smoking should be avoided and weight reduced in cases of obesity.

(v)   Artificial insemination by the husband (AIH) is used, making use of the split ejaculate technique when the man's sperm count is low, but not too low for consideration. This technique involves collecting the sperm produced by masturbation. The first half of the sample is placed in one container, the rest in another. The first half, being richer in fertile sperm, is then inseminated into the woman's vagina.

Artificial insemination by donor (AID) is widely used to help fertile women who are married to infertile men, but it is important to remember that while this technique (described later) can fertilise the woman, it is not a treatment of male infertility. It is a means for a couple to have a child, using another man's sperm, where the man is infertile.

In-vitro fertilisation can also be used where there is a low sperm count, and the woman also has a fertility problem. Either the first half of a split ejaculate, or donor sperm, can be used to fertilise an egg outside the womb.

Unexplained infertility

Despite the current advances in medical and surgical treatments for infertility, there are still many people who undergo extensive tests for infertility and for whom no conclusive reason for infertility is ever found. 'Unexplained' infertility may be diagnosed if the woman is ovulating regularly, has open fallopian tubes with no adhesions, fibrous growths or endometriosis (scar tissues from the womb lining found outside the womb). The man must also have normal sperm production. Intercourse must take place frequently, particularly around the time of ovulation, and the couple must have been trying to conceive for at least the previous two years. Under these criteria, about 10 per cent of all infertile couples would appear to have unexplained fertility problems. This proportion would probably fall to about 3 per cent if thorough laparoscopic screenings and other tests were carried out.[2]

(a) UNEXPLAINED OVULATORY PROBLEMS

Luteal phase abnormalities are perhaps the most important of all causes of 'unexplained' infertility. The luteal phase is the part of the female menstrual cycle that follows after an egg has been released from an ovary. After releasing the egg, the follicle (tiny bag) in which it was contained within the ovary goes on to become the corpus luteum (yellow body). This produces the hormone progesterone, which is essential to the preparation of the lining of the womb to receive the fertilised egg. Progesterone from the corpus luteum sustains the embryo in its first seven weeks of life, after which the placenta takes over production until delivery.

Several things may go wrong with progesterone production. The rise in output may be too slow; the level may be too low; or the length of time over which it is produced may be too short.

Possible causes In general these are not able to be conclusively ascertained, but some tentative explanations have been advanced:

(i) The abnormalities may be the result of problems with the two gonadotrophic hormones. Lower levels of FSH seem to be responsible for the production of smaller amounts of progesterone by the corpus luteum. Lower LH levels, too may be responsible for a failure to develop an adequate secretion of progesterone. The ratio between the amounts of LH and FSH appears to be critical to progesterone production.

(ii) Luteal phase defects may sometimes be caused by abnormal levels of the hormone prolactin.

Investigation

(i)   Endometrial biopsy. Samples taken from the lining of the womb are examined.

(ii) *Blood samples.* These are taken on different days after ovulation. The level of progesterone within the blood can be measured, and the progesterone output monitored. Similarly, blood levels of prolactin can be checked (see page 26).

Treatments

(i)   *Clomiphene.* This may be useful in helping to restore adequate secretion of FSH and LH. Luteal-phase abnormalities, and abnormalities in the development of the follicle, or in the timing of ovulation, may be helped by this drug.

(ii) Progesterones. These can be given as injections or vaginal suppositories, to help luteal-phase abnormalities. Synthetic 'progestins' should *not* be used; they have an anti-progesterone activity, may cause the corpus luteum to die, and are also broken down into male hormones within the body. This could adversely affect a developing embryo.

(iii) *Bromocriptine.* This drug may successfully reduce high levels of prolactin.

(b)   BLOCKAGE OR ABNORMALITY IN THE REPRODUCTIVE ORGANS

These problems are the result of structural or mechanistic deficiencies in the woman's reproductive system.

Possible causes

(i)   There may be a defect in tubal motility which prevents the successful passage of the egg down the tube.

(ii) Abnormal levels of hormones called prostaglandins may interfere with the passage of the egg in the fallopian tube. These hormones are responsible for making the muscles of the tubes contract. (High prostaglandin levels are usually associated with endometriosis – see page 28).

(iii) The egg may be released from the follicle, in which it develops, before it is properly mature.

(iv) A few cases of unexplained infertility may be due to the persistent production of abnormal eggs. These eggs may have a deformed structure, or chromosomal abnormalities. (The chromosomes are the genetic 'blueprint' for the transmission of characteristics to any fertilised embryo).

(v)   Sometimes eggs are produced, and mature correctly within the follicle, which goes on to become a corpus luteum. But the corpus luteum does not burst and release the egg. Thus the eggs are trapped inside the unbroken corpus luteum.

Investigation and treatment   Though it may be possible to diagnose the abnormalities described above, by the use of the various tests already mentioned, most of the abnormalities are not really treatable within the limits of current medical expertise. However, recent advances, for example, with in-vitro fertilisation, may well change this prospect.

(c)   OTHER 'UNEXPLAINED' INFERTILITY PROBLEMS

(i)   There is some evidence that some sperm, though adequate by normal definitions, is unable to penetrate the woman's egg in order to fertilise it. There appears to be a correlation between this type of infertility, and the inability of sperm to penetrate the egg of a hamster from which the outer coating has been removed. The zona-free hamster test is producing some interesting research results. This test can explain at least some cases of 'unexplained' infertility.[3]

(ii)   Infection by certain disease particles has been shown to be responsible for some cases of unexplained fertility. A disease particle – T-strain mycoplasma – may be present in numbers that are not enough to show up in a clinical examination, but which nevertheless may cause infertility. A group of couples who had been infertile for five years, with no obvious cause, were treated with a broad-spectrum antibiotic to clear up any possible infection with T-strain mycoplasma. Twenty-seven per cent of the women conceived within five months.[4]

(iii)   Psychosexual problems may possibly be the reason for a small proportion of infertility cases.[5] A couple may be unable to consummate intercourse, or they may have sexual intercourse too infrequently. Psychosexual problems may sometimes be helped by professional counselling.

(iv)   Stress may also have some significance in infertility. The whole hormonal cycle, with its delicate adjustments, is controlled from the brain, which responds to its immediate environment. Disturbances in the chemical balance within the brain would therefore affect both behaviour and the hormonal control mechanism.[6] This is an area which, however, needs further investigation.

We have described briefly some of the more common problems of male and female infertility, their possible causes, and their investigation and treatment. In the next chapter we shall look at some medical techniques in current use which, though they offer hope to the childless, are to a certain extent controversial, as their use could challenge our current understanding of the nature of society, and how it works.

4

Some controversial techniques

There are several medical techniques in current use or in process of being developed, that offer hope to the childless in their quest to have a child of their own, but whose use is to a greater or lesser extent controversial. The controversies surrounding the techniques go beyond purely medical issues, and involve legal aspects and moral/ethical questions to do with general understandings of what society should be like, and what should be permitted within a particular society.

We will give a brief description of these techniques before summarising the main arguments relating to their use and development. Many of the issues are discussed in the Warnock Report, first published in 1984.[1] This report made several recommendations for government action to be taken for the control of the use of the techniques, and for controls on related medical research. However, no indication has as yet been given as to whether the government intends to incorporate the main recommendations into any composite Bill to go before Parliament.

(a) Artificial insemination by donor (AID)

This technique, now widely used, involves the collection of sperm, by masturbation, from a fertile donor who is not the husband or regular partner of the woman who is to receive the sperm. The semen, preferably collected fresh, but sometimes held frozen, is then placed into the vagina, cervix or womb using a syringe, or special insemination cap or, on occasion, a contraceptive cap or diaphragm. It can be done at home, or at a clinic under a doctor's supervision, or with the help of a specially instructed nurse. When a cap is used, it can be left in place for a short time to help bathe the cervix in sperm, thus improving the chance of conception. The technique can be used where the man has little or no sperm, or where he has a genetic defect which should not be allowed to pass on to any offspring. It can also be used by women without a partner, and by lesbian women. Donors of sperm are usually selected, and as far as possible their race, blood group and physical characteristics matched with those of the woman's infertile male partner. As far as is practicable, the medical and genetic backgrounds of donors are also assessed. The technique itself is perfectly legal, although there is some legal doubt as to the legitimacy of the child at birth. There are no legal guidelines given to registrars of births, and as a result, most parents indicate that the regular partner is the natural father, or give no named father on the birth-registration form. When donor insemination is carried out with the male partner's consent, it does not constitute grounds for divorce.

Because there is a third party, a stranger, involved in the fertilisation of the woman, there are some ethical problems connected with the use of donor insemination. Some religious groups oppose the technique on the grounds that it is unnatural, or that it weakens the structure of family life. Others argue that it is a God-given way for a woman, married to an infertile man, to have a child and to found a family without breaking the marriage vows. With both views, a question of conscience is involved. The individual couple considering donor insemination are, whichever way they decide, sacrificing the interests of one of the partners. If the decision is against donor insemination, the interests of the fertile female partner are sacrificed; if the decision is for donor insemination, the man may be giving his assent in order to compensate his wife, despite his own feelings about the use of another man's sperm to fertilise his wife. Although the technique is relatively simple, and in increasing demand, all couples contemplating undertaking it should go through the ethical issues carefully before coming to a decision to accept it. Recently, in view of the problem of the possible transmission of auto-immune deficiency syndrome (AIDS), a screening process has been introduced to prevent carriers of AIDS from donating sperm.

Members of the National Association for the Childless who took part in a survey on attitudes to donor insemination in 1982 strongly supported the use of the technique in appropriate cases.[2] Donor insemination was preferred to adoption as a solution to infertility, as it was seen to offer at least one partner the chance to have their own child. Secrecy was, however, seen to be necessary, indicating a general concern over the unresolved legal questions on legitimacy; and also a fear of possible public shame if the man were known not to be the natural father of his wife's child. The possible effects on the child, in receiving such knowledge, might also be a factor in the desire for secrecy. There is a feeling amongst some concerned professionals that the maintenance of secrecy could be detrimental to the family life of those who have children who were conceived with the help of donor insemination.[3] However, it is generally regarded as a fairly simple, straightforward technique whose continued use in appropriate ways is not detrimental to the functioning of a society, provided that it can be regulated sensibly. This may be because, by itself, donor insemination as a technique has a limited number of possible applications.

This is not the case with the technique to be discussed next, *in-vitro* fertilisation (IVF), which appears much more threatening to our current perceptions of how society should operate. Though (IVF) (fertilisation in a glass dish) offers a means for a couple to have children who are legally and biologically their own (an advantage for a couple over donor insemination, where a third party takes part in the conception), the social ramifications which could follow from extensions of the use of the technique are enormous. They call into question our present understandings about the nature and development of society. Further uses of donor insemination in relation to extensions of IVF will be discussed in this next section.

(b) *In-vitro* fertilisation and related techniques

Several related techniques will be briefly described and discussed in this section. These are:

> *in-vitro* fertilisation
> egg donation
> embryo donation
> surrogacy
> freezing and storage of human semen, eggs and embryos[4]

Inherent in all research connected with these techniques is the question of whether it should be permissible for research to be undertaken on human embryos.[5] This is a very fraught area of the controversy, which will be briefly alluded to in a separate section after the techniques have been described and discussed.

1. IN-VITRO FERTILISATION

This is commonly known as the 'test-tube baby' technique and is used in cases where the woman's fallopian tubes are blocked or deformed. It may also be appropriate where the man's sperm does not penetrate the woman's egg because of hostile-immune factors (see page 29). It is sometimes used in cases of 'unexplained' infertility, or with women suffering from the effects of endometriosis (page 27). It can also help cases of low sperm count or motility. The man's sperm is introduced to the egg outside the woman's body, in a small glass dish (*in-vitro* or 'test-tube'), and an embryo is formed. The embryo is then returned to the womb, where it grows like any other foetus.

The technique is still in an early stage of development, and success rates are generally around 30 per cent.[6] There are a number of necessary stages involved. A ripe egg has to be collected by laparoscopy from an ovary. The laparoscopy must take place during ovulation, so tests must first be performed to ascertain that ovulation is occurring. A sample of the man's semen is also required, ready to fertilise the egg as soon as it is removed from the ovary. The egg is placed in a special fluid in a laboratory glass, and the sperm (in the man's semen) is then added. The resulting interaction between the sperm and the egg is observed through a microscope. If fertilisation takes place, the embryo has to be returned to the womb (embryo replacement). If the embryo plants itself in the womb lining, it will develop in the normal way, just as if the egg has been fertilised in the fallopian tubes.

A very recent development of the technique, in its early stages of use, is gamete intrafallopian transfer (GIFT).[7] An egg is taken from the ovary and immediately transferred to the fallopian tubes. At present the egg is fertilised by artificial insemination, but it is likely that the husband's sperm will eventually fertilise the egg naturally after the operation. This form of IVF offers hope for those women whose egg-bearing follicles in the ovaries open to release an egg, but whose egg fails to pass into the fallopian tubes (there must, of course, be no damage to the fallopian tubes). It is a much less dramatic form of intervention than the classic IVF form, and omits the actual 'test-tube' stage.

The IVF technique by itself is relatively uncontroversial, though a few call it 'unnatural'. The main difference of opinion amongst practitioners of IVF is probably over the number of eggs that should be fertilised and returned to the woman's uterus. Several multiple pregnancies were achieved in the earlier stages of the use of the technique, and there is a general feeling amongst the medical profession that multiple births (beyond two) are not generally in any woman's medical, psychological or social interests.[8] There is also a feeling on the part of some of the public and doctors that those selected to undergo IVF should conform to certain social and/or moral standards of suitability. A woman who has, for example, children by a previous marriage, has undergone voluntary sterilisation and is living with a man to whom she is not married may be considered by some to be an 'unsuitable' candidate for IVF. However, it is difficult to know whether this is primarily an argument about social views of morality, or whether it is about the choice of criteria for selection of IVF candidates where there are limited public funds available to carry out the operation.[9]

2. EGG DONATION

This is a form of IVF where a woman donates an egg so that a second woman may carry, give birth to and bring up a child which the second woman regards as her 'own'. It is suitable for those women who cannot produce an egg or whose ovaries are inaccessible. The egg is usually fertilised *in-vitro* with the sperm of the second woman's partner, and is then implanted in her uterus so that her pregnancy can proceed normally from then on. It is assumed that the resulting baby will belong to the woman who receives the egg. A baby was born by this technique in Australia in 1983.[10]

The arguments for and against this type of technique are similar to those for and against donor insemination, in that there is a third party involved in the conception, and one of the nurturing parents of the subsequent child is not the biological parent. The Warnock Report recommends acceptance of this technique under similar terms as those of donor insemination.[11]

3. EMBRYO DONATION

Embryo donation is like egg donation, except that both sperm and egg are donated. Thus there are four people involved over the various stages of the process. Two are the man and woman who donate the sperm and egg, the third is the woman recipient who will carry and give birth to the child. The fourth is the recipient's partner who becomes the nurturing father, but like the recipient, the nurturing mother, he is not the biological parent of the child.

The arguments against embryo donation are similar to those used against donor insemination and egg donation. In addition, neither party has any biological relationship to the child, so that it has been suggested it be considered a form of pre-natal adoption.[12] The Warnock Report gives guarded recognition to this form of treatment, seeing it as likely to be suitable for a very small number of couples. It should be treated in the same way as egg donation and donor insemination, with safeguards for the nurturing parents and the child.

4. SURROGACY

This is a possible way for a woman to have her 'own' child without giving birth. The more common form of surrogacy is where the fertile male partner's sperm is inserted into the womb of a third party, a woman who has agreed to carry and give birth to the subsequent child, and then to hand the baby over to the man and his infertile partner, to be in all respects the couple's 'own' child. Or the sperm may be mixed with the surrogate's egg *in-vitro* and returned to the womb. This form of treatment is suitable where the woman of the partnership can neither conceive or carry an embryo, for example, a woman who is post-menopausal, but whose husband is fertile. This form of surrogacy is sometimes called partial surrogacy, to distinguish it from the other possible form, full surrogacy,[14] where the male partner's sperm is mixed *in-vitro* with the female partner's eggs, which are then placed into the uterus of the surrogate who will carry and give birth to the child. The child will be the biological child of both the nurturing father and nurturing mother. This form of fertility treatment would be suitable for a woman who could produce eggs in her ovaries, but who had no uterus.

In practice, all the arguments about surrogacy relate to the partial form, where the egg is obtained from the surrogate, as the technique is relatively simple to carry out. Surrogacy evokes very strong negative feelings on the part of large numbers of the public, and amongst many professionals as well.[15] To conceive and carry a baby in the womb for another couple for nine months is physically and emotionally an awesome task, and there are likely to be very few women who would undertaken this for purely altruistic reasons, so financial inducements are usually offered to surrogates.[16] With or without the exchange of money, the couple wishing to obtain a child by this means are in a very vulnerable position, as even in countries where surrogacy is permitted by law to operate, no court seems at present likely to rule against a surrogate who decided to keep the baby she had given birth to.[17]

In the UK the major argument against partial surrogacy is probably a widespread feeling of abhorrence at the idea of the child who is subsequently born being exchanged for money. 'Buying' a child in this way may be considered similar to slave-trading, wife-selling, and dubious forms of private adoption where the adopting parents pay a third party who has obtained the child for them. The motivation of the surrogate may also be regarded as suspect, in that she is considered to prostitute herself (in a general sense) by demeaning the sanctity of 'motherhood'; on the grounds that no normal mother could part with a child she has carried in her womb in exchange for financial reward.[18]

Interestingly, where a surrogacy arrangement takes place between relatives, this may be regarded by some as a legitimate use of the technique. A fertile woman who acts as surrogate for her infertile sister may be considered to be doing it out of love and compassion.[19] Also, there is some support for full surrogacy, as both the adopting parents are the genetic parents of the child they will bring up.[20] The only involvement of the surrogate is in the 'leasing' or 'lending' of her womb.

However, it must be stressed that opinion is generally heavily against surrogacy, and in the UK any arrangements made for commercial surrogacy are illegal.[21]

5. FREEZING AND STORAGE OF HUMAN SEMEN, EGGS AND EMBRYOS

As scientific knowledge has advanced, it has become more feasible to store semen, eggs and embryos by freezing them in liquid nitrogen. Thus it is possible, for example, for several eggs to be taken from a woman's ovaries, some used straightaway for her IVF operation, and the rest stored so that she can go through the operation again at a later date if the first operation fails. This, in principle, would be regarded as a welcome scientific advance.[22] However, other possibilities are also opened up by this technique. A man who knows he is dying of cancer may have his semen stored, so that after his death his sperm may be artificially inserted into his wife's womb, and she will then give birth to her and her late husband's child, possibly several years after her husband's death.[23]

Thus all kinds of possibilities are opened up, which could threaten current understandings of family life and of how society should operate. Current legislation in most countries is inadequate to deal with such questions as whether an embryo is or is not a person, whether it has rights of inheritance, who in fact it belongs to. Many hospitals where modern infertility treatment takes place have some kind of ethics committee, which tries to make appropriate decisions as to what should and should not be permitted in general, and in individual circumstances. But the whole area is so controversial, and it is such a new area of human experience, that it is very difficult for those working in the field, and those advising them, to know the most appropriate decisions to take.

(c) Embryo research

Since it has become possible to fertilise eggs and sperm outside the womb, and to store any surplus embryos, the opportunity for research into and on embryos has been presented to scientists. This kind of research is attractive to scientists for many reasons. It can help to further understanding of ways of overcoming infertility, preventing miscarriage and helping doctors and scientists to understand more about many other aspects of conception and childbirth. It can also enable research which might help scientists prevent or find a cure for several very terrible medical conditions such as cystic fibrosis and muscular dystrophy. It may become possible to determine at a very early stage whether a pregnant woman is carrying a gravely handicapped foetus, and enable her to decide whether to continue the pregnancy.[24]

However, there is also the possibility that new forms of human being could be produced from this research, and some kind of 'brave new world' of brain-washed human drudges or evil geniuses be let loose on the world.[25] And embryos could also be used to test drugs, or as organs for 'spare part' surgery in transplants.

Thus there are reasons to be cautious about permitting complete freedom to those who wish to experiment on embryos. But there are also many who feel that research into embryos is wrong in principle. Many of those who do not support embryo research base their opposition on religious principles of reverence for life, and the use of embryos for research is for them a form of murder, the embryo at its conception being considered to have the full rights of a human being.[26] There are others who would support some modified form of embryo research, limiting it to the period when the embryo is known to have no form of nervous system, and thus to be unable to experience pain.[27] However, it is difficult for experts to agree on a particular stage of development beyond which embryo research should not be permitted. The Warnock Report settled for the arbitrary limit of fourteen days, which is the latest stage at which identical twins can occur, and well before the development of the nervous system.[28] The Warnock Report recommended the setting up of a system of controls on embryo research, but as yet the government has announced no plans to set up any system or form of control.[29]

Concluding remarks

As was said in the introduction to the previous chapter, the survey of medical problems concerned with infertility was not intended to be comprehensive, or to go into great detail on all aspects of investigation and treatment. Readers are referred, through the notes, to more detailed treatments in other books. What we hope has emerged is that there is a broad variety of treatments available. It is likely to be the case that, for many infertility patients, the main problem is in gaining access to the centres where the most up-to-date treatment is available. For those whose problem is 'unexplained' infertility, it is suggested that there is a fairly good chance of there being a medical explanation to their problem if they have the opportunity to go through an intensive treatment programme. The implication seems to be that infertility patients may need to assert some of their rights as consumers of the health services if infertility treatments are to be available to the same standard in all areas. But it must be understood that whether certain treatments become more widely available is more than just a medical and/or financial decision. Certain of the more recently developed techniques pose a series of legal, ethical and social questions which need to be looked at by society as a whole.[30]

Another purpose of this description of the medical aspects of infertility was to act as a background to a broader view of childlessness as a comprehensive problem affecting all the major aspects of the life of an infertile person or couple. The medical description will be needed as a counterbalance to the many myths and misconceptions that have sprung up about the nature and causes of infertility, which have helped to perpetuate inaccurate and damaging stereotypes of the childless.

5

Myths and misconceptions

The previous chapter attempted to show that infertility is primarily a medical problem. Though individuals undergoing treatment for infertility may be very distressed about their situation, there is very little to suggest that infertility is a psychological state of mind.[1] Even where infertility seems to be 'unexplained', there is likely to be some possible medical reason, which could be discovered with the help of new or more sophisticated medical treatments.

This, unfortunately, is not how infertility appears to the majority of the general public. In some parts of the country infertility may still be a 'taboo' word, too awful even to be considered or discussed. In other areas, infertility is recognised, but seen as a 'personality defect' – there is something wrong with, or lacking in, a man or a woman who cannot start a family; and this character deficiency is vaguely perceived as the primary contributing factor to childlessness. Though based on ignorance, the myths which are spread about the childless can still prove very harmful to those who are on the receiving end of what may often appear to be malicious gossip. Someone who has discovered his or her infertility may also find that there is little support to be had from those he or she ought to be able to trust. Sometimes ill-informed ideas about childlessness are not made explicit, but act as some kind of underlying influence on the way the childless are perceived.[2]

Common myths about infertility

Possibly the most influential myth about infertility or childlessness is that it is a woman's problem; and a man cannot be in any way 'at fault'. This is socially legitimated where there are severe social penalities for any man who admits that he has failed to make his partner pregnant. In some societies traditional folk wisdom may make it unthinkable that anyone should believe a man could be responsible for his wife's failure to produce a child. In some parts of the world, even giving birth to a girl is a cause of shame to a woman, and she may have to go on producing babies year after year until she has given birth to a boy. Only then can she be regarded as a full member of her society, and be allowed a rest from the bearing of children.

It would seem reasonable to suggest that this myth about infertility as a female problem has ancient origins, perhaps to do with the fact that it is women who give birth. Where there is a lack of education on the matter, it is possible that the link between sexual intercourse and pregnancy is not perceived (one does not always need to look as far as an exotic tribe to find evidence of this ignorance). The patriarchal nature of many societies would also help to reinforce the myth that a woman is responsible for fertility and pregnancy. Where the social status of a man is considered higher than that of a woman, it would be counter-productive for men to admit to something that would lower their own status in the eyes of other men, if the 'blame' could legitimately be shifted onto the woman. Sometimes this shifting of 'blame' is a result of a traditional acceptance of the very different roles assigned to men and women within a particular social group. Again, it must be stressed that one does not need to look too far from home for evidence of this. From time to time letters are received at the NAC office from women who cannot proceed with fertility investigations because their partner refuses to undertake any tests, or even in some cases to accompany the woman to the hospital or clinic. Yet these men may be perceived by their partners to be extremely fond of children.

In more reasonable environments, it is possible that the myth is a result of the fact that in most cases it is the female partner in a relationship who visits the doctor first in any enquiry about infertility. A survey by David Owens and Martin Read in 1979 showed that with 70 per cent of couples who completed a questionnaire, it was the woman who contacted the GP first. Twenty-five per cent of couples went to their GP together, and only 3 per cent of men initiated enquiries.[3] The authors of the report on the survey suggest a variety of reasons as to why this pattern should emerge so clearly. They disregard the point that women generally consult their GPs more often than men, as the frequency of women visiting first for enquiries about fertility was much higher than the percentage visiting for general medical problems. Owens and Read suggest that women may be more concerned with children than men and, despite recent trends towards job equality, women are more likely than men to be responsible for child rearing, and to have been conditioned to accept the role of 'mother'. There may also be an assumption that the wife is at fault, possibly through the belief that the wife's reproductive system is more complex than the man's; there is a greater probability that something will go wrong with the woman's reproductive system. Also, women's gynaecological problems are more apparent; while men with subfertility problems may have been producing what looks like a perfectly normal ejaculate.

Owens and Read also bring up the question of general ignorance about male medical fertility problems. They suggest that most medical evidence indicates that in at least 40 per cent of cases of involuntary childlessness, the male will have a contributory medical problem. They base this figure on estimates by Robert Newill in 1974 and John Stangel in 1979. Andrew Stanway also quotes this figure; and Naomi Pfeffer and Anne Woollett suggest that the figure is about 35 per cent.[4] The most general estimates, including those made by the above authors, show figures which suggest that the problem is as likely to lie with the man as the woman, and that there is also a third category of infertility problem where both partners are involved. Thus there is very little to support the view that infertility is a 'woman's problem'. But there is evidently a great deal of ignorance among the general public; and a need for greater publicity and education on the essential nature of infertility as a medical problem likely to afflict both sexes fairly equally. It is only in recent years, however, that it has become possible to discuss the issues rationally, and in some parts of the country, to be known to be infertile still carries a great social stigma.

A second myth that is still perpetuated is that the childless are as they are because of their psychological make-up. Elliot Philipp and Barry Carruthers have suggested that less than 5 per cent of all infertility patients are likely to be infertile for psychological reasons; they stress that infertility is a very distressing condition, which needs careful psychological support.[5] What the public seem to mistake is the direction of the problem. They observe individual childless people in states of distress or depression, and assume this is the cause, rather than the result, of infertility. Also there is usually a general revulsion when some childless woman behaves in a dramatic way, and steals a baby from a pram. This rare occurrence, which is usually treated with some leniency when the poor woman is taken to court, can be taken as evidence by the public that all childless women are unstable, and that society and babies should be protected from such people. At a more mundane level, those who have children may be totally unable to comprehend the reaction to their children from those who do not have children of their own. When a childless person has to withdraw from all contact with children, as a safeguard against exposure to too much emotional stress, this is taken to mean that the childless are peculiar in some way. In her excitement about her own baby, a mother may find it hard to believe that there are those who do not share her own joy. As the childless seem to have so little in common with others in normal social interaction and group membership, people find it hard to think of them as normal, unexceptional members of society.

A third, still fairly common, myth is that the childless couple are rather cold, unfeeling, people, who are seen to live in homes that are neat, tidy, well-furnished, and hostile to the more messy kind of life-style to which most people with children are forced to adapt. It is almost as if tidiness is now considered proof of a self-centred materialism. There is the rather sad story of the childless woman who was sitting in her garden, and she heard two of her neighbours (and, she thought, friends) discussing her over their fence. This woman had undergone intensive treatment for infertility over a period of three years, and had finally been told by the consultant that the main reason for her fertility problem was that her husband's sperm were not strong enough to penetrate to her fallopian tubes. She was feeling very depressed, and unsure how her husband would be able to accept this information; he had gone very white and silent when told by the doctor. She felt that the whole of the last three years had been spent battling to have a baby. Both the neighbours she heard talking had, she felt, been kind and understanding, and very patient when she felt she just could not bear to see their children, particularly the new baby next-door-but-one.

What she overheard was mean and rather thoughtless gossip. The one said to the other that 'she had been to the hospital yet again today'.

'I don't know why she bothers', said the other. 'She'd have to be a lot more perky than she is, with children about. She'd cry at the drop of a hat and never manage them.'

'Do you think so?' said the other. 'I don't think she really wants them at all. Look at their house, all neat everywhere like a posh hotel room. I think she just goes through the motions for him really, and gets upset about him wanting them. She's a frigid type, you can tell the way she goes round all uptight. I bet he gets it up her only when she wants.'

The woman crawled along the lawn and into her house, so as not to show that she was there.

Yet another myth is that childlessness is the result of a sexual disorder. The previous chapter on the description of infertility as a medical problem has shown that infertility is likely to be the result of sexual difficulties only in a minority of cases. Philipp and Carruthers suggest that failures in the effective performance of intercourse will account for between 5 and 10 per cent of all cases of failure to conceive, and that self-confidence and practical advice are more important than psychiatric help in solving the problem.[6] Common sense also suggests that the majority of childless couples are likely to be no different from other couples in their capacity to perform sexual intercourse. It has been suggested that, with those couples who have intercourse infrequently, there is more likely to be a failure to conceive, as the likelihood of intercourse taking place at the right time is thereby decreased.[7] But this is something which is not easy to prove.

It is likely that there is some general confusion over the meaning of the terms 'infertility' and 'virility'. Each is supposed, in the uninformed mind, to imply the other. Infertility has already been defined as a medical condition, but what is virility? Is is a high sperm count in a man, or a stronger than average need to have sexual intercourse with a woman, or to have it more frequently than usual? Is it related to perceptions about the size of the man's penis, a larger penis being considered more masculine? The word 'virile' implies possession of the characteristics of a man (from Latin *vir*, man). One current dictionary definition does include both procreative power and manly vigour within the several given meanings.[8] Thus it would seem that, in their general meanings, fertility and virility are in some way linked. But again, as with the myth about the psychological inadequacy of the infertile, there is a confusion about the direction of the relationship between the two terms. One does *not*, of necessity, imply the other. If it did, the heroes of most American soap operas would be paying huge maintenance bills for the hundreds of children they must have fathered in the course of their weekly or nightly adventures (they never ask if the woman is taking the pill).

In fantasy, the vigorous aspect of 'virility' is exhalted as a virtue. In reality, the man who is seen not to have children is considered lacking in masculinity or virility. There is the story of the shop-floor worker in a motor-components factory. He was in the factory lavatory one day and overheard a conversation between two of the men he worked with. They had been talking about their children, and the one went on to say 'Old Ron', (he was 35 at the time), 'hasn't got no kids, poor bugger'. The other man saw it rather differently.

'Well,' he replied, 'you can tell really, he can't give his missus enough stick, can he?'

'Why not?' the other asked.

'Well, most of them blokes are a bit nancy'.

The other then said, 'Yes, I've always thought he weren't one of us'. The man went home, and asked to change his job in the company, he felt so humiliated. His wife had severe endometriosis, and had had several unsuccessful operations to remove the scar tissue. She also felt her husband was too demanding sexually, and his sperm count was around 100 million, more than adequate for conception to take place.

One myth which, fortunately, is slowly dying out, is that infertility is incurable. In the face of the medical evidence to the contrary, it is surprising that this myth still holds ground. But it seems characteristic of many people that they build up their world picture from an amalgam of the experiences of those they come into contact with, ideas they have inherited from family, and childhood experiences. Three or four cases of an event or occurrence are often sufficient for them to form a generalisation of potentially enormous magnitude. Statistical evidence cannot compete with this first-hand experience. Due to the difficulties involved for many people in obtaining satisfactory medical treatment for infertility, it is unfortunately possible for people to genuinely believe that infertility is incurable. The local hospital may have a very poor record, as a result of a lack of facilities for fertility treatments, or a low level of interest in the related fields of treatment. Or a couple may decide to stop treatment, leaving their friends convinced that here is another example of the incurability of infertility. The stress brought about by treatments can also lead to depression and loss of interest in the sexual side of a relationship, thus perpetuating the likelihood of childlessness. In the absence of a social climate which favours open discussion about fertility, it is difficult for most people to judge correctly, from observation of the experience of others, whether infertility can be 'cured' or not. Conversely, those people who keep very quiet about their own medical investigations, and then, say, have a child by donor insemination, may never have to reveal that there is or was an infertility problem. It is hoped that exposure to more accurate information, reinforced by responsible treatment of the subject in the media, will cause this myth to die out altogether in the not-too-distant future.

Some misconceptions about childlessness

Many of the myths described in the previous section can be attributed to a general lack of knowledge or awareness of the problems of childlessness. With greater effort given to education of the general public on the issues involved, some of these myths would slowly begin to disappear. Misconceptions are, however, a result of a very different set of affairs. The common misconceptions about childlessness are based upon an individual or group awareness or understanding, and not upon a general ignorance. The *myths* are reinforced because people fail to think too deeply about the problem; the *misconceptions* are the product of the thinking of those who are often well-informed, and altruistic.

Over the last few years there has developed a growing awareness, particularly but not exclusively, among younger people with a fairly high level of education, that the world is going through a crisis of a kind that humankind has never experienced before. Unless the problems of this crisis are dealt with as a matter of urgency, there is a danger of the world disintegrating into brutal anarchy or a succession of oppressive dictatorships. Two particularly worrying features of the current world crisis are the enormous population increases likely before the end of the century; and the inequitable distribution and utilisation of the world's resources, particularly its irreplaceable resources. There is an awareness that it is the rich countries of the 'North' or 'West' that have greatest access to, and control over, the use of these resources. An individual born into one of these societies consumes far more of these resources than someone in the 'East', 'South', or the lesser developed countries. Yet these latter are the countries with the fastest growing populations. Thus the stage is set for bitter conflict, unless there is some readjustment of the present world system in the interests of all, rather than just the interests of the richer countries.

One effect of this realisation has been an emphasis, in Western countries, on an individual's responsibility in limiting the size of his or her family, in the interests of society and of the world. In general this has acted for the common good, and has also fitted in with currently held views about a woman's right to freedom of choice as to whether or when she has children. However, the concentration on the necessity for population planning and control has, indirectly, had an adverse effect on the position of the involuntary childless. As well as having to cope with the effects of widespread ignorance about their condition, they are increasingly being called upon to justify their decision to pursue lengthy or expensive fertility treatments in their quest to have their own child. It is somehow considered immoral or irresponsible of them to be so preoccupied with their own personal, even selfish, need for a child, when the world is so manifestly unable to provide adequately for the majority of the children it already has.[9] The childless are somehow made to feel guilty for daring to ask for help with a problem which is 'not really a problem' at all, but the result of too much concentration on their own needs, to the exclusion of the needs of everyone else.

This criticism should not be dismissed out of hand.[10] It is undoubtedly true that the impending crisis, which some have attributed to the world population explosion, will only be averted if there is an understanding among individuals and nations that what happens in one part of the world has direct consequences for the rest of the world. The rich, as well as the poor, do have to make responsible decisions about the number of children they should have. And a country may decide to have a national population policy as regards the upper and lower limits within which it wishes to stabilise the size of its population. China, for example, has decided that its population problem is of such magnitude that it must be controlled by regulations. Each couple is allowed to have one child only.[11] Singapore, by giving incentives to small families and encouraging the better-educated women to produce at least two children, hopes to have a stable population of 'good' intelligence by the year 2030.[12]

Having said this, however, the question remains as to whether it is right, or even appropriate, that childless couples should be made to feel guilty for wanting their own child or children, particularly if they would need the cooperation of medical science for the woman to become pregnant. There are two answers to this. The first is that, despite the social problems caused by population increases, an individual does see his or her need for a child as personal, and of great importance. For most people, having a child is considered an essential and very much valued experience in life. Children are regarded as giving great pleasure, and they contribute to the quality of family life.[13] The right to a child is also enshrined in the United Nations Charter of Human Rights.[14] This would suggest that the government of a just society does have some responsibility for ensuring that, where possible, a couple should be able to have a child or children of their own. The needs and wishes of a population do have to be taken into account in policy decisions.

The second answer to the question as to whether the childless should be made to feel guilty for wanting a child in an overcrowded world, is that, in pragmatic terms, the number of children likely to be born as a result of the pursuance of medical treatments will not have a perceptible influence on the population figures. It takes at least 2.3 children per family for a population to remain at the same level.[15] The majority of the childless would want two children at the most. Many would be extremely satisfied with one child. And in the UK, in particular, where the population is not predicted to increase, there is not the same urgency to prevent wanted births as there is in some other countries. Arguments about the inequity of resource distribution between the rich and poor countries will not be solved merely by balancing out population statistics so that the population of the developed countries has to decrease to make up for the increase elsewhere. It is the amount of resources consumed by each person that will make the difference, not increases or decreases in the birth figures.

Thus it can be seen that there is not a particularly strong case, in terms of national or international needs, for the childless to be deprived of the opportunity to have children. And in wanting a family they are no more or less selfish than the majority of people who regard having children as a natural consequence of a marriage or long-term partnership.

Another misconception which has grown up over the last few years is that the childless, by seeking and undertaking expensive medical treatments within the National Health Service, are depriving the 'genuinely sick' of the resources needed in high-priority areas of treatment. The childless are made to feel guilty for asking for help, because they are continually made aware that where there is competition for scarce resources, their own needs cannot be expected to take priority over the needs of the acutely ill, and those who would die without the availability of emergency treatment. The childless feel doubly guilty because they know that they themselves might one day need emergency life-saving treatment, and this makes it even more difficult for them to argue the case that greater priority should be given to fertility treatments. Again there is a misconception behind the arguments involved. The childless are only 'depriving' others of treatment if the concept of a fixed health budget remains central in one's thinking. If this is the case, the more one person has, the less there is left for others. But the national budget consists of much more than a health budget. If the national wealth is looked at as a whole, and the national interests also looked at as a whole, it becomes possible to see that there exists a set of national priorities which determine how important each area of spending is in relation to any other area of spending. There are several areas of national spending which are quite controversial, for example the defence budget, and in almost every country in the world this budget is a source of contention.[16] The childless have to argue their case, not as attempting to deprive the sick of vital resources, but as demanding adequate consideration from the national budget as a whole. All of this looks extremely simple when spelt out, but it is surprising how people become conditioned into limiting themselves to a small area of operations, and try to balance unsatisfactory solutions one against the other, rather than questioning whether they really are restricted to the one area of operation.

This chapter has attempted to show how the childless are handicapped socially by being the victims of two very different sets of views. The myths still perpetuated about the childless portray them as socially deviant, or as in some way abnormal. Because of some deficiency of character they are condemned to remain childless. Although the medical facts suggest that this stereotype cannot be true for the majority of the childless, the myths linger on as a result of general ignorance or misunderstanding. The misconceptions described in the second section of the chapter imply, in contrast to the myths, that it is the childless themselves who are ignorant, and in need of education, to make them more aware of their social duties and their responsibilities towards the world as a whole. The childless, therefore, see themselves as downgraded by two completely different sets of criteria, and there is much to suggest that they are a very vulnerable group as a result of the conflicting pressures put upon them. The next chapters will show the extent of that vulnerability through a survey of the responses of some of the childless to the medical, social and personal aspects of the experience of infertility and childlessness.

6

Infertility – the endless treadmill? Medical aspects

Anyone who decides to undergo treatment for an infertility problem or to obtain a child by other means is likely to be in for a hard time. There may be some whose cause of infertility is quickly diagnosed and successfully treated. And there may be a few who apply for adoption, are accepted without delay, and subsequently receive the baby they have always wanted. But, for the majority of the childless, the experience of actively seeking a solution is fraught with difficulty at almost every stage. It is as if they are condemned to a life sentence walking a treadmill. Some never quite recover from the trauma. Ten, fifteen years after the first realisation of a problem they are still on the search, long after they have been told that 'nothing can be done for them, and isn't it about time they started thinking of alternatives?' Others are fortunate in eventually being able to have their own child, or a child through donor insemination or adoption. But the majority have to make a decision at some point to stop the search, and to seek for fulfilment in life in other ways. In this some are more successful than others.

The experience of undergoing infertility investigations is a traumatic and unnerving experience for most people. One problem is that, despite the optimism of some medical specialists, there is no guarantee of a successful outcome. Uncertainty surrounds the whole experience, and a feeling of desperation begins to set in if a satisfactory result has not been achieved within a reasonable time. In addition, a couple undergoing examination and treatment may, as a kind of insurance, be applying for adoption at the same time and, for the majority of the childless, there can be few experiences more demoralising than being told that an adoption society has closed its lists, or that they are ineliglible to apply. But perhaps even that is preferable to being assessed and turned down. The couple are not only under pressure from the effects of fertility investigations and worries about being accepted as adoptive parents;

THE INFERTILITY TREADMILL

THE MEDICAL SIDE

Medical facts
e.g. Husband has a zero sperm count.

Socio-medical facts
e.g. The tendency for couples to postpone having children leads to a rise in infertility.

THE SOCIAL SIDE

Social facts
e.g. Abortion and changing attitudes to illegitimacy mean fewer babies available for adoption.

Social barriers
e.g. The low status of infertility in the NHS discriminates against those who cannot afford private treatments.

Society
e.g. The childless feel alienated from friends who have children.

Attitudes of society
e.g. An adoption agency considers the childless unsuitable for older child adoption.

PERCEPTIONS AND FEELINGS OF THE CHILDLESS

SOLUTIONS

Medical barriers
e.g. Fertility services are poor in some parts of the country.

Medical profession
e.g. Consultant tells woman she is infertile in brutal unsympathetic way.

Attitudes of medical profession
e.g. GP is against women over 35 having fertility treatment.

they are beset by a host of other pressures, from those who are expecting them to produce children, and from those who make them aware that one can only be a full member of society by becoming a parent.

> *Like blossom*
> *that beaming face*
> *Fulfilled –*
> *Gladdened by thoughts*
> *of being*
> *Normal at last*
>
> *No longer*
> *that strange look*
> *Reflecting*
> *a cruel past*
> *But smiling*
> *Receiving*
> *Her son – her chance*
>   *(Anon.)*

The childless feel under threat from all sides. Sometimes they keep their feelings to themselves; at other times they are overwhelmed and burst out with complaints against the medical profession, social workers or their relatives. The childless who are aware of their infertility are very isolated. They are turned in upon themselves in their isolation, and are likely to go through several very negative experiences related to both the medical and social aspects of their problem. This is illustrated in the diagram on page 48. This shows the central core as the perceptions and feelings of the childless, rather hemmed in, like a womb. They can escape from this womb to a world of medical facts, barriers and attitudes which appear to attack them, or to the world of social facts, barriers and attitudes. They may eventually reach a solution; if they are lucky, the one they wanted, but only after much suffering.

Why is the experience of infertility portrayed so negatively? The answer is simply that, for the hard core of the infertile who do not find any immediate answer to their problems, it *is* a negative experience. Support for this view comes from the literature on infertility, and from a reading of the many thousands of letters that are sent to the office of the National Association for the Childless.

MEDICAL FACTS

Let us look at the diagram on page 48, and relate it to the perceptions and feelings of the childless towards medical facts. By a medical fact is meant some kind of diagnosis or finding by a medical specialist, about which it is very difficult for the layman to disagree. Medical facts often have a horrid kind of finality about them. For example, a husband is told that his sperm count is zero. For this there is at present no successful treatment. Or a man may have had mumps as a child, which in his case has left him infertile. Then there are the more complex cases, like the problems of a husband who has two grown-up children from a previous marriage, but cannot fertilise the *in-vitro* eggs of his second wife. He learns that male fertility falls off in the late forties to fifties. For the couples who have to come to terms with the finality of the medical diagnosis, and its effect on their future hopes, there is likely to be great distress and unhappiness, even if the eventual outcome is that they achieve a child by other means. A man with adopted children wrote that, despite the fact that his wife was very happy with the children, he himself could not really believe that he was sterile. He was still rather shocked about it.

Sometimes the confrontation with infertility seems tragic, as in the case of a woman whose only conception had been when her first marriage was breaking down, and she had a termination because at the time she felt unable to care for a child adequately. Another sad case is the woman who was physically disabled in an accident:

> I am partially disabled. I had a serious motorcycle accident four years ago, in which I fractured my spine, and it left me paralysed from the waist down for a year, but now thank God I can walk on crutches.

She is inquiring about adoption. Or there is the woman suffering from Hodgkins disease, having a hard time, but still interested in having a baby.

> I was first diagnosed as having Hodgkins Disease at the age of 19 and received radiotherapy. Further treatment followed two years later and again four years after that. Three years later we began trying to start a family. After two years of failure I got an appointment at the infertility clinic and at the same time began to look into the possibilities of fostering and adoption. Unfortunately this coincided with a recurrence of Hodgkins. Therefore, instead of embarking on fertility tests I found myself undergoing chemotherapy. This ended last February and my periods are gradually returning to normal. I have basically come to terms with being childless, my main priority is staying well. On the other hand, if there is hope for us I would like to explore it.

There is another type of medical fact which by definition seems out of place here, but is just as much a fact as a chromosome defect or an early menopause. This is the 'cause not known' fact. It is every bit as depressing as a negative diagnosis. With the latter the loss of fertility can be mourned, but 'cause not known' sentences a couple to a kind of limbo: 'We have not been given a reason for being childless. As the years go by I find no reason very difficult to accept.' Is there a cause, which the doctor has not been able to determine, or is there nothing wrong with them, and if so, why has the woman not conceived? Is it stress? And so they go round in circles, becoming ever more distressed. Much depends on the way the specialist handles such a couple. One doctor tries to sum up the situation from the practitioner's point of view:

Having been closely involved with infertility for 15 years or so, I increasingly marvel at the ease with which some women become pregnant (in spite of all the contraceptives) and at the other end of the scale, I increasingly despair at the number of women who desperately want to become pregnant and who, in spite of all the treatments, do not become so.

This honesty is sometimes difficult for the childless to deal with, because they may, in their determination to have a child, treat such a statement as admission of incompetence, rather than as a statement about the limits of medical knowledge.

MEDICAL BARRIERS

Medical barriers, in general, are medical situations which prevent the infertile from achieving their objectives. They do not have the finality of medical facts, but they are often great sources of irritation and frustration to those seeking treatment. There are several common areas of dissatisfaction. First is the length of time that fertility investigations take. Most letters to the NAC office start off in a very similar way:

We have tried for a baby for six years with no success, during which time, I must say that doctors have been very unsympathetic and we've yet to meet anyone who is even interested in our problem. It has been a constant struggle throughout. Doctors have to be pushed and pestered into doing tests. Why, we don't know.

I am writing to tell you how thrilled we are at the birth of our baby son on June 30th, after about five years. I now understand about everyone else's trials and tribulations.

It is not uncommon for periods of ten years or more to be mentioned. Another area of complaint is about the side effects of drugs. A woman on Ovran 30 hormones found that her hair was falling out. Another developed an ovarian cyst through taking Clomid, and was later told that she did not need to take it anyway. Here is a description of some of the effects of Clomiphene:

> I find there is a discrepancy between your notes on Clomiphene and what I have been prescribed: now on my seventh cycle with this double dose I am experiencing serious side effects: dizziness, nausea, headaches, skin rashes, swollen breasts and depression, and have been so upset as to warrant a visit to the doctor.

There are other unpleasant drug combinations:

> Since seeing him, we have found a cause for our problems, and that is, that I don't ovulate. Simple you might say, but finding the right combination of drugs is very different. I started on Clomid, with an HCG injection and Ethinyloestradiol, but couldn't tolerate it. I then went on to Tamoxifen plus injections. The side effects, if no one points them out to you, can almost drive a couple apart. I put on weight, we argued constantly, I threw things (frequently at dinner) at my husband. I spent days locked in the bathroom screaming at him, and all the time he has stood by me. My moods could change at the least little thing, even that it was raining and I couldn't put the washing out.

A third medical barrier is the lack of priority accorded to fertility treatments under the National Health Service:

> We decided to have AID. We were put on the waiting list and told that we should have to wait about a year and that treatment should begin no later than June of this year. We are still waiting (Sept). We have been told that they cannot tell us when the treatment is likely to begin due to shortage of staff etc. as a result of cutbacks in the National Health Service.

Infertility treatment such as *in-vitro* fertilisation and donor insemination are regarded as 'spectacular' and non-essential, detracting resources from routine, more essential medical treatment. In this connection, people living in certain areas of the country, particularly in rural areas, may not have access to up-to-date facilities for fertility treatment. Even in large hospitals with gynaecological departments, fertility may be part of the same section as abortions and sterilisations.

Sometimes, unfortunately, the childless suffer as a result of medical incompetence. One woman, after ten years of treatment, went to a

Harley Street doctor, who showed her that her husband had a sperm abnormality and could never make her pregnant. Here is another case:

> I was seen at a clinic in the local hospital. I had examinations and then was admitted for a laparoscopy which showed endometriosis and I was given various tablets and treatments. None worked. I then had a second laparoscopy and again the same treatment. Then four years of my notes went missing from my file and from then on things went from bad to worse. I was given injections daily (Perganol) and even this course was not completed. I was then given a six-month break and told to return in September. Upon my return the intention was again daily injections of Perganol. Upon telling Doctor X of all this he has told me there was no need for the second laparoscopy, my tablets were set on wrong courses – three months instead of six months – and the Perganol I should never have had at all and should have been warned of various symptoms which could have been caused.

As the result of a new treatment programme, this woman is now ovulating – after five years of investigations that brought her no benefit.

Sometimes medical facts and medical barriers are linked. For example, a woman with a serious adrenal disorder and asthma became pregnant after fertility treatment from a specialist. However, her GP was in disagreement with this, as he did not think she was fit enough to carry through the pregnancy. Sadly, he was right and she subsequently had a miscarriage.

ATTITUDES

When we turn to the attitudes of the childless towards the medical profession, two sources of distress emerge clearly. The first is that the childless feel strongly that they should not be treated in the same room as those undergoing miscarriages, abortions or sterilisations. To mix with pregnant women is also a most distressing experience:

> He suggested a laparoscopy, which I had last month. What really upset me was I had to go to the maternity hospital and was in the ward with threatened miscarriages. Very distressing. We found the hospital completely insensitive to infertile women, especially when they give you AIH in the same clinic and at the same time as pregnant women are seeing the doctor.

Another woman writes:

> When I went into the hospital to have the scan I was very scared and

worried. I was put into a room with three other girls. The first woman was pregnant and all she did was moan that she wished she wasn't. The second girl already had five children and had been sterilised after the last, had then remarried, wanted another child and this was the only way. I thought she was mad.

One hesitates to ask what was wrong with the third woman.

These experiences serve to confirm what many of the childless feel, that their problems are insignificant in comparison with the medical problems of others. Obstetrics and gynaecology cover a wide range, and it is understandable that medical staff, when faced with life-threatening situations, will feel that non-urgent cases must take second place.

For the last two years I have been attending a small local hospital. I have, however, not been happy at this clinic, just being sandwiched between maternity and gynae problems. I have also been seen by several doctors, thus losing any continuity. I feel that there is very little interest in my case and that they have many more 'serious' and pressing cases to deal with.

A better solution might be separate infertility clinics, as happens in some areas.

Secondly, for any childless woman undergoing treatment, the worst moment is likely to be when she is told that she has come to the end of the road with medical tests, and that she should begin to think of alternatives. It cannot be easy for any doctor to give bad news to a patient, and it is possible that even the most sympathetic doctor would be unable to convey the finality of his or her verdict to a childless woman, in any way that would soften the blow. Just being told is traumatic:

I think the hospital I attended for five years has given up on my ever conceiving. The nurse more or less said 'There is not much more we can do for you now, Mrs. Jones.' I did feel shattered, and only wished there had been someone at the hospital to talk to.

Some are unable to believe the doctor could be right.

So we asked about operations to clear the tubes, but she shook her head and said, 'Well, you have your health now – what's more important?' What a question!

Then she turned to my husband and said she was not very happy with his sperm motility – something we had previously been told was all right. After asking about drugs to improve it she said, 'Oh, no, there's nothing we can do for that.' But the crunch was, after our silence after being told both my tubes were blocked, she thought it best we started seriously thinking about life without any children. We cannot get over the attitude – no talk of don't worry, we will do everything we can – it was goodbye, there's nothing we can do for you – but there is, there's the test-tube process ...

In the absence of full information it is difficult to judge the rights and wrongs of this case, but there does seem to be a need for some kind of counselling, when a doctor feels that a couple are finding it difficult to take in what is being told them. This couple had received a shattering blow, which would force them to consider a complete life re-appraisal; and they were not at all equipped to begin this.

Sometimes a couple do not have to wait long for a verdict.

In October my husband and I began fertility tests when a longed-for pregnancy did not occur. The first result showed that my husband had an extremely low sperm count. The specialist wrote to say no further treatment was available and advised us to think about alternatives.

Most specialists in male fertility would regard the results of only one sperm test as unreliable. This woman did in fact have a baby at a later date. Among many of the childless there is the feeling of a lack of any sympathy on the part of the specialist, and on a few occasions the specialist is considered arrogant or patronising. The 'good' specialists often seem to be those who help a couple achieve a child. If they do not, they are likely to be seen as baddies, which is, we suppose, understandable.

Just as the childless have strong feelings about members of the medical profession, so doctors and others have strong feelings about some of the childless. Sometimes a GP is in disagreement with a couple's pursuit of treatment for infertility.

Now I am on a mixture of Clomid and Tamoxifen and injections which I can tolerate reasonably well. The next step is Pergonal, as I still don't ovulate even on these drugs. We will have to pay for this as well as all the drugs, as my local GP has come to a decision that he can no longer help us.

Another GP thinks a couple are wasting their time:

I have been in touch with my local Contact about private clinics and she has told me that facilities are bad in our area. My GP has said that it would be a waste of money as he thinks there is nothing wrong with me, only tension.

The woman has been on fertility drugs for a hormone imbalance. Disagreements between the specialist and the GP may, in certain cases, have effects that could not be foreseen.

I was told at the hospital by the pharmacist that I would have to go to my own doctor for any further prescriptions of the Bromocriptine drug.

When I approached the GP, who was not my usual doctor, he also refused to give me any more prescriptions as he said something like 'I don't want to be signing a death certificate for you.'

So I was unable to get any satisfaction from my own doctor. Although I am 36 years of age now and have never conceived, I thought my own doctor would go along with my own wishes to 'try anything' to give me a chance to get pregnant.

The other Saturday I was so depressed I tried to kill myself by taking tablets and drinks. I ended up in the General Hospital.

Time may, or may not, validate the GP's assessment. How much treatment a patient should be given requires a finely balanced decision, though many of the childless find that they have to push for further tests to be done. What is more worrying, at a more general level, is the attitude of infertility specialists, implicit or explicit, concerning the nature of women in general, or infertility patients as a special group. Specialists who do everything in their powers to help the childless achieve their objectives, may be conveying, to future generations of medical practitioners, damaging stereotypes of women which may prove difficult to eradicate, and which influence the way in which a doctor approaches a patient. One gynaecology textbook summarises infertility thus:

Inability to conceive is a denial of woman's dominating instinct, and some degree of neurosis must be expected. The patient is likely, in her eagerness, to accept any form of treatment, and the gynaecologist must consider at each step whether further intervention is justified.[1]

There probably are women who behave in the way described, and for whom 'neurotic' is an appropriate medical description, but it is alarming to think that a young male gynaecology student goes into his specialist field armed with the view that all his female fertility patients will be neurotic.

Infertility patients have also been described as 'selfish'. In a description of an otherwise advanced and caring approach to fertility treatment, a specialist, in describing the work of his infertility clinic secretary, writes:

> The present secretary is a relatively young grandmother who has returned to part-time secretarial work in the hospital. Infertility patients become very selfish and self-centred – perhaps more so than any other kind of patient – and tend to telephone to demand attention not only while attempting to become pregnant, but also once a pregnancy has started.[2]

Again there are likely to be childless women who fit this description. But perhaps 'selfish' is not a very appropriate or helpful word. 'Demanding' and 'needy' are perhaps better, although 'demanding' does have certain negative connotations. The infertile are 'demanding' because they have a need, which is urgent and impelling, and they have placed great faith in the medical profession to satisfy that need. They are also fearful, and under great pressure from relatives and society to achieve pregnancy and childbirth.

There is much more that could be said on many of the issues mentioned in this chapter, and the main points are dealt with in more detail in other chapters. However, the main point of this chapter has been to illustrate the kind of dilemmas and problems experienced by the childless as they attempt to grapple with the complexities of the medical system in trying to find an answer to their fertility problems.

It has been shown that there is a large degree of dissatisfaction among fertility patients with the health service provisions in this area of medicine. Many people find it difficult or impossible to obtain appropriate treatment and the overwhelming impression given is that infertility is the Cinderella of modern public medicine. This is understandable in the light of the current political philosophy of public health provision. Doctors must do what they can with fewer and fewer resources. But there is the risk of pushing infertility treatment out of the public sector altogether, so that only those who are well-off will be able to achieve what people in all social classes normally take for granted – a child of their own.

7

Infertility – the endless treadmill? Social aspects

We have seen how important medical facts, barriers and attitudes can be in hindering the childless in their search for a solution. Until fairly recently there was an alternative available to them – adoption. But the social changes of the last twenty years, that have brought benefits to many, often appear to the childless to have been at their expense.

Social facts

Two important social facts have changed things for the childless. The first was the passing of the 1967 Abortion Act, which has resulted, over the past few years, in about 135,000 fewer babies each year being born than are conceived.[1] One cannot argue that all of these babies would have been available for adoption, as many women who conceived an unwanted child might have felt, under circumstances where abortion was illegal, that they should keep the child born to them, or hand it over to relatives. But the likelihood is that there would still be many more babies available for adoption if the 1967 Act had not been passed. As it is, fewer than 4,000 babies and children a year are adopted by non-relatives.[2] This is not to argue that abortion should consequently be made illegal. Even among the childless there are many who feel that women should not be forced to give birth under all circumstances, and that the right to choose to give birth is a principle that should be upheld. This is, however, a very controversial area, both among the public at large and among the medical profession. One doctor, on being asked, by a childless couple, why single women who had abortions were not counselled to give birth and hand the baby over to the childless, replied that he did indeed do this, but the women refused, preferring an abortion.

The second major change over the last twenty years has been in attitudes towards illegitimacy, and the gradual acceptance of the one-parent family as a de facto unit of society. Gone are the days when single women felt compelled to give birth in secret and to give the baby up for adoption. Many single women now deliberately choose to give birth, without being in a long-term relationship with a man. Although the lot of many one-parent families is still a very hard one[3], the existence of the Welfare State does help prevent the starvation and destitution of the 1930s, and fewer people part with their children in the hope of giving them a better chance in life.[4] However, the absence of children for adoption has led some desperate couples to seek children by very dubious means, such as surrogate mothering which is carried out (illegally) for a fee. In choosing this, the childless lay themselves open to exploitation by the unscrupulous. Surrogate mothering (where a woman carries a baby for another woman) is generally condemned by society, but it serves as an illustration of the lengths to which some childless couples will go to obtain what they feel is not unreasonable in a society which still sets a high premium on having children as a pre-requisite for full social integration. After all, as Prince Charles is on record as saying, after watching the birth of his heir, 'It's a very grown-up thing to happen to you'.[5]

The chart on page 48 will show that there is a category of fact which is medical in effect, but social in origin. The tendency for women, for social reasons, is to postpone having children until they are past their most fertile years.[6] In theory the answer should be simple – women should have their families at a younger age, but this would have social repercussions, especially for women. The women who at present tend to want children at a later age are those who are interested in establishing themselves in a career first. It is difficult enough for women who have worked, and then had time off to bring up a family, to re-enter their careers or jobs at a later date. If women are to give birth earlier, before they have had much relevant work experience, or before starting a career, it would be that much more difficult for them to enter a career or job structure at a point where they would be equal to men who are their contemporaries. At present those women who have reached a certain salary level in their profession can afford to make adequate child-care arrangements, if they wish to remain in their careers. This is unlikely to be the case with the 21-25 age group. Thus, though it is obviously preferable for women to give birth at an age when they are most fertile, there is a danger that they might thereby face more discrimination in attempting to find employment.

Social barriers

The social barriers faced by the childless, as opposed to the social fact of the non-availability of children for adoption, are fairly narrow in scope. The first barrier is to do with the ways adoption societies impose requirements on would-be adopters in order to restrict the number of applications for the very few babies available. Although some of these regulations act to ensure that children are placed in the best available homes, a large number of the childless are automatically excluded from making an application.

The main regulation by which they are excluded is the age barrier imposed by the majority of adoption societies. It is interesting to note that a large number of members of the National Association for the Childless are in their thirties. Some have spent many years undergoing medical treatment for infertility and do not reach a decision to try for adoption until they are too old, by most adoption agencies' standards. Others happen to have married late, and even though their infertility may be quickly discovered, there is not enough time left to adopt. The fact that the older couple may feel their greater life experience makes them ideally suited to bring up a child is held to be of no account. It is possible to appreciate the reasons for preferring younger couples. The sheer physical and emotional energy required to cope with the demands of a very young baby are very evident. However, it is a pity that by the imposition of age limits, most older couples are excluded from the adoption of babies and very young children. In the population as a whole, a proportion of women in their late thirties and early forties do give birth and bring up their children successfully. Other adoption societies operate by closing their lists from time to time, or only accepting people resident in a certain area. These somehow seem kinder ways of turning down would-be adopters, although the end result is the same.

Because of the scarcity of babies, even a couple who are assessed, and considered suitable to be adoptive parents, may lose out, because by the time a baby is found for them their situation has changed. There is the case of the couple who were due to receive a baby the day after the wife was rushed to hospital for a hysterectomy. The husband informed the adoption service and as a result the baby was given to another couple. As the wife was now over forty, they were automatically crossed off the list. One can imagine the anguish of this couple, the futility of their recriminations against one another, and their desperate need for help with their pain.

Older-child adoption is sometimes suggested to the childless. In theory this ought to be an answer to the problems of the childless who are not eligible to apply for babies, and in some cases it works very well. But for the majority of the childless it is not usually appropriate. We were told by one woman how she had gone to an adoption meeting organised by her local social services department, and the social workers had described in detail the children who were on offer, so to speak. She quickly realised that all the children were unusual, they were mentally or physically handicapped, or black, or a complete family, including older children, who needed to be placed together. One wonders why she had not known before that it would be like this. But it was a terrible shock for her. At half time she disappeared to the ladies toilets for a quiet cry, and found them full up with women crying over the same disappointment as hers.

The only other likely source of babies and young children is from overseas, and some couples have succeeded, against overwhelming bureaucratic opposition, in adopting a baby or young child from a developing country. This is costly, both in time and money, and only to be recommended for the most robust. It takes a certain kind of dedication to carry it through successfully, and requires people who are sensitive to, and tolerant of, cultural differences.

Adoption is one area fraught with social barriers. The other is the failure of the NHS to provide some of the more promising new treatments, with the result that only the better off can afford to have them privately. Many people write to the NAC office, unable to go further with their fertility treatments as they are working class, or unemployed, or live a long way from London. A man from York wrote:

> We are hoping to have AID in London, but do not know if we will be able to afford any expensive tests. Do you have any ideas on what our chances of success are? We will only be able to go once a month because of the distance (and expense involved).

Test tube babies are beyond the means of most people:

> I can wait a while longer for my baby, because the test tube price is too high for us working class people. Why £3000 for a test tube, but only £100 for a private abortion to end a life?

As was said, overseas adoption is expensive:

> Carol sent me some papers (a copy of the application for adoption of children from Bangladesh). I know Kevin and I would like to send off for details ourselves but haven't any money to go ahead with trying for a baby from overseas.

Sometimes people wonder if they are being exploited in the private sector of medicine. One might question whether a woman who has had donor insemination for four years without results is helping to line the practitioner's pocket. The lack of controls over donor insemination is not to the advantage of the childless, and it is hoped that this situation will be regularised. But it is not always easy to control the private sector and not particularly desirable that the childless should be forced to use it as a result of NHS deficiencies.

Attitudes

When one comes to the attitudes of the childless to society, and society's response to them, the situation is fairly complex, as the childless feel under threat from a variety of sources. They react towards those close to them – parents, brothers and sisters and friends who have children. They react also towards 'society' in the abstract, but when one looks at this 'society' one finds two contradictory strands. On the one hand, the society of traditional values enshrined in the concept of the family (now nuclear) is urging them to conform by having children. On the other hand the women's movement is saying that childbearing is only one of many options open to women. Some feminists also suggest that what is called the maternal instinct is not innate. Elizabeth Badinter argues, from a historical study of childbearing practices in Europe, that women have been culturally induced to see themselves primarily as mothers.

> A review of the history of different forms of maternal behaviour gives birth to the conviction that maternal instinct is a myth. No universal and absolute conduct on the part of the mother has emerged. On the contrary, her feelings, depending on her cultural context, her ambitions, and her frustrations have shown themselves to be extremely variable. How then can one avoid concluding, even if it seems cruel, that mother love is only a feeling and, as such, essentially conditional, contingent on many different factors? The feeling may exist or may not exist; appear and disappear; reveal itself as strong or weak; be focused on one child or lavished on many. Everything depends on the mother, on her history and our History. No, there is no universal law in this matter, which transcends natural determinism. Mother love cannot be taken for granted. When it exists, it is an additional advantage, an extra something thrown into the bargain struck by the lucky ones among us.[7]

Although this viewpoint is helpful to those who doubt their ability to cope successfully with being a mother, and to those who have not been fulfilled by motherhood, it is not generally helpful to the childless. It appears to undermine the legitimacy of what they are doing – trying by any means possible to achieve a child of their own; yet the strength of their desire in no way measures their capacity to be a good mother. Thus, the childless appear to fail by two sets of criteria, conformist and non-conformist.

Many of the reactions of the childless are directed towards those people who are in close contact with them. Some feel that having a child will strengthen an already strong and loved family. 'I have had a few months break again from treatment whilst we had my mother-in-law dying of cancer at my brother-in-law's home. Sadly she died in February without ever seeing our much wanted child.' Others find difficulty in showing the appropriate interest when a relative becomes pregnant. 'How does one explain to a pregnant relative that I am just not interested in her baby or her?' For some the experience is very bitter:

> Sister Sharon, now aged 21, has a 6 months old baby whom she farms out at least 3 full days, plus one evening a week – she's been married 20 months. I found out today, via my aunt, that Sharon is underway with adoption proceedings – yet she can have children. What hurts most is that she and all the Cornish lot know about it. Yet *we* didn't ever know anything about it.

Friends in general are a very difficult experience for the childless to handle. The childless do not know whether to talk about their problems, and be pitied, or to keep silent and be misunderstood. If a friend becomes pregnant, the childless woman may feel extremely hurt. When the friend's baby is born the friendship may change, as neither woman has the same interests: 'But it can be upsetting that for most other people of similar age, their problems seem to be connected with their children and, of course, their lifestyle is very different.'

Workmates are not always as sensitive as they might be. For the childless, the ritual of ex-mates proudly bringing their new baby into the office for the ritual 'coos' and 'isn't he/she beautiful?' can be very painful:

> Because our new neighbours are retired it is hard even to make friends, and just have someone to talk to, because as you know the girls at work are as hard as nails, I don't really think they know what the word understanding is – especially when someone brings in their new baby.

One NAC member, when depressed about this, had a different feeling:

> The low was a deep depression and near breakdown of my mental stability. This was caused by people's stupid and unfeeling remarks, particularly with people I work with in close contact every day, and who all have children (naturally). This is why I ask for particular help

in this matter, as my recent reaction, held under control, is to grab them by the throat.

Friends who really care for someone who is childless often try to make things easier by belittling the satisfactions of having children. This is well-meant, but is sometimes misinterpreted by the infertile, who would willingly experience the agonies of parenthood. This is perceptively expressed in the following poem:

> *N.A.C.*
> *What's that?*
> *O Jack,*
> *Sit down and eat your tea.*
> *A National Association for who?*
> *Poor Sue,*
> *Is that you?*
> *Childless, I mean.*
>
> *Still, never mind,*
> *You should have some of mine,*
> *You'd soon find*
> *You'd wish you hadn't,*
> *It's all the noise –*
> *Quiet boys!*
> *The mess and the toys*
> *That would ruin your lovely house.*
>
> *You've got a nice job,*
> *A dog,*
> *and Bob.*
> *What more could you want?*
>
> *You see,*
> *I fell so easily,*
> *I only planned to have three,*
> *But now I've got more than I wanted.*
> *It doesn't seem fair,*
> *Really Clare!*
> *Don't stare;*
> *She's not used to all you children.*
>
> *I never gave it a thought*
> *that there really ought*
> *to be an Association just for your sort.*

I suppose I was too busy with the family.
Well, Sue,
There's so much to do,
It's been nice seeing you.
Call again after I've had the baby.

JENNIFER TERRY

Some NAC Contacts who subsequently have a child find it difficult to convey their news to childless members. The Contacts fear the effect it may have. One member who became pregnant received hostile letters from other childless members.

It is distressing to some of the childless to live on estates where there are large numbers of families with young children, or to live in a small traditional rural community. On estates, the childless women are automatically excluded from all the regular meeting places where young mothers make friends – toddlers' groups, playgroups, mother and baby clinics, school gates and parks. In small communities, there is a great deal of gossip, and traditional expectations that a young married couple ought to produce a child as soon as possible.

Beyond family and friends, the feeling of the childless may be very negative indeed. They may express strong feelings about social workers from adoption societies. As one woman wrote:

Coming back to the social worker though, I do feel it is entirely true what we were all saying at the Conference, that they really are loathe to give you a reason, and to say the least, opinionated, and it seems so wrong that the recommendation is by the one person in such an important decision.

It seems one does not actually have to apply to adopt to sense one is not wanted: 'It appears impossible to adopt a baby in this country (and indeed the literature we have received on adoption seems aimed at making one feel guilty about wanting to do this).' Some childless women turn against abortion counsellors and those who have abortions:

Why can't they set up counselling for women who want abortions – and let them know what it's like to be childless, and help see how they could help childless couples by having their baby and giving it up for adoption. If they could only realise what it would mean to a childless couple.

It seems incomprehensible to some of the childless that abortion should be favoured over adoption as a solution to the problem of unwanted babies. The solution is obviously not as simple as suggested, but for those who do not support abortion, it seems that an injustice has been done to the childless.

On issues such as donor insemination it is interesting that, although the childless see themselves as an isolated suffering group, they may tend to be supporters of a conservative view of society, as based on the nuclear family with two parents and children. In a survey carried out by David Owens,[8] over half the childless respondents were against donor insemination being given to single women, and well over half against it being available to lesbians. In the survey, remaining childless was rated the least acceptable solution to the problem by over half the respondents.

The childless express their feelings about society, and in return society has feelings about the childless. Many are very sympathetic, but they are unable to show their sympathy in a way that does not cause more hurt. Parents cannot always accept that they have an infertile son or daughter. They have their own needs to fulfil:

> We are currently getting over the hurdles of letting our parents know that there is no hope. We have never really told them the whole story, particularly the AID part, but recently I was able to tell my mother-in-law the general situation.
>
> It was at the time the Princess of Wales had her baby and they were staying with us for a few weeks. The day the announcement was made, the overwhelming news coverage hit a nerve deep down. I am sure the same thing happened to many other childless couples. I suddenly found myself unable to hold in my feelings any longer and sobbed uncontrollably for half an hour. I felt the heartbreak of years flooding out and I know it was healing. My mother-in-law came up to the bedroom, not knowing what the matter was. As she comforted me I was able to talk. Needless to say she was desperately sad but she did her best to soothe me and said something that I think showed great wisdom. She said: 'You will never be happy until you have finally given up the idea that there might be a chance'. I know she is right.
>
> My own mother is far less understanding. A few weeks ago she actually said to me: 'If you don't do something about it, I'm going to advertise for some grandchildren.' The outburst was also due to the fact that my brother had 'murdered' one grandchild – his girlfriend had an abortion. I could not even be angry. She knows I have been going to the clinic for years. I could not spill tears for her. I have none left.

It is often hard for parents to accept the idea that one of their children is infertile. They may suffer when their own friends start to boast about their grandchildren. Like their children, they too feel that they are excluded from an essential stage of life's experience. Families do not always appreciate the needs of a woman who has struggled to become pregnant:

> *Our Sylvie lives in her flat at the top of our street*
> *But she couldn't be bothered to use her two feet*
> *During the whole of my pregnancy she called only once.*
> *The rest of our tribe all live within one mile*
> *I missed them all – it was quite a while*
> *The short bus ride costs only 8 pence*
> *Yet they never came near*
> *And no-one wanted to hear of my fears.*
> *On the day I aborted they all gathered round like ghouls,*
> *Young Lesley aged ten sat with big eyes like an owl,*
> *But their interest was now too late*
> *The baby was dead – will this be my fate? ...*

(Anon.)

The plight of one infertile woman had a very direct effect on her friends:

I try to put on a brave face for family and friends – fortunately no-one else I know has had this problem and in fact quite a few have decided to commence their families earlier than planned for fear it could happen to them as well.

But in general there is a very uncomfortable silence on the subject. It even permeates the women's movement. Naomi Pfeffer and Anne Woollett, writing a feminist account of the experience of infertility, have this to say:

These feelings of isolation were accentuated for us because, as feminists, we had expected to be able to talk to other women, to be able to discuss our infertility within a feminist context. But we found the taboos and silence just as strong within the women's movement. This made us very angry. It denied the reality of our experience.[9]

In their concern to help women obtain release from what Lynne Segal calls the 'nightmare of illegal abortion'[10] and the fear of sex, feminists have not realised that the needs of a different, increasing group of women are not being covered.

If correspondence and phone calls to the NAC office are anything to go by, social workers are another group who are often unsympathetic to the childless, or who appear to alienate them during adoption enquiries and assessment. Of all the ways of acquiring children, this is probably the most difficult now, and it is likely that tensions arise on both sides because of this. As one woman said, 'You have the feeling that the local authority can hold your future in their hands'. Which, of course, they can do in this respect. Sometimes the reasons given by an adoption society for turning down a couple reveal underlying attitudes antagonistic to the childless and their ways of coping with their problem. A man who worked in a training centre with adolescents, and a nurse in a special baby care unit were given the reasons for their lack of success:

> Then to be turned down as unsuitable for adoption! Reasons – 'That to place a child into our relationship would put that relationship at risk'. Secondly, 'wondered if Neil could cope with a child during adolescence'. Thirdly, 'wondered if I had accepted our childlessness as the panel couldn't understand why I had chosen to work in a special baby care unit at our local maternity hospital, they thought perhaps I was being a little too maternal'.

There may be reasons not being revealed here by the adoption society or by the couple, but the implication is that any childless or single man or woman who works with babies or young people, is doing it with some dubious motive, to do with the satisfaction of unacceptable personal needs. This couple subsequently adopted a child through another agency, but for most, a negative decision is final.

> We are still having no luck with adoption. I rung up the social services, who still said that the sub-committee's decision was final, and that the lists were now closed again anyway.
> It puts a terrible strain on a marriage, doesn't it? We are still finding it hard not to blame each other.

Suffice to say that there *are* good sympathetic social workers in many areas, and that the job of assessment is done with fairness and compassion. But to be turned down for adoption is a crushing blow, and it may take a couple a long time to recover their self esteem.

One effect of bringing to the attention of the public the special needs of the childless has been to spotlight the more unusual and often socially unacceptable ways of obtaining a child. The media are very keen to castigate anyone who tries, for instance, to find a surrogate mother. The couple can then be called 'selfish', because they should be helping the world's 'needy' children. Anyone who has tried to adopt a child from overseas will be able to vouch for the fact that most of the world is not particularly keen for its children to be helped in this way. Social workers will also bear witness to the difficulties involved in helping an older child who has been in care for many years. This view of the childless is only another version of 'Eat up your crusts, because of the starving children of Africa, or India, or You-Name-It'.

Suffice to say, not all media accounts are of this type, and many childless couples have been portrayed sympathetically. It was too much for the parents of one childless woman, however, when they discovered that she and her husband had been interviewed by their local press for an artical on infertility:

Today my mother phoned at 7.30 am in a state of extreme agitation, backed by a multi-voiced mutually agreed 'choir' in varying stages of hysteria. The reason for all this is that I have committed a terrible crime by talking to a local newspaper reporter about my husband and I, in that we are childless, and mentioned NAC.

'How on earth can we hold our heads up at work when that comes out?'

'You haven't mentioned any of us? We don't want to be connected with *that* sort of thing.'

'How do you think we'll feel if anyone does recognise you as of our family?'

It takes courage to maintain one's viewpoint against such an onslaught.

Some of the reactions presented in this chapter have appeared rather extreme. Obviously, many childless people and their families and friends manage to reach some sort of accommodation between their different viewpoints. Love and affection moderate the disappointment. But what this chapter has tried to show is that social changes have led to a drastic worsening in the traditional situation of the childless, and that since they appear, by comparison with yesteryear, to be much worse off socially, they are bound to react as most deprived groups eventually do. They do this in order to draw attention to their need, in the hope that society will begin to understand their plight, and try to do something about it.

8

Infertility – the endless treadmill? The feelings and perceptions of the childless

We have looked at the childless in relation to the medical and social facts and barriers with which they are confronted, how they respond to the medical profession and society in general, and how these two in turn respond to them. But the real drama lies elsewhere. For the infertile, another world exists. Some of it is confided to the staff of the NAC office, but for every confidence given one must assume a lot left unsaid.

Women, for it is mainly women who write or phone, describe a great variety of experiences and feelings. Many are common to the experience of infertility. There is the feeling that no-one else in the world has quite the same problems:

> We have been trying for a baby for nearly three years now, we've had lots of problems, at the moment we both feel we are the only couple to have problems. I know we're not, but at the moment we don't know where to turn.

There are the mood swings and the depression that settles when the monthly period arrives as usual. There is the destructive effect of lovemaking. Sometimes a woman turns against her own body. Here are some extracts from a diary:

> … In a few months it will be our fourth anniversary – our fourth anniversary of trying to have a baby, I mean.
> … I *am* pregnant. I'm sure I am. Life is great. I can't take in how great it is. I can't stop smiling, and can't sleep. I'm so full of energy. What's the tiredness you read about in pregnancy books? I could go on forever. Haven't told anybody yet except Miriam and Giles.

... (3 days later). An unspeakably horrible day. I've cried all day long. I feel as if a real baby's died. When we got in tonight, I went mad and smashed a milkbottle, but what I really wanted was to smash me, to die in the most horrible gory way possible and punish my stupid body.

Time passes too quickly, and nothing changes: 'I have many (too many) childless years behind me.' It is difficult to make any realistic plans for the future: 'I find if very difficult to try and sort out anything in the future, e.g. changing jobs or moving house.' The marital relationship may come under serious pressure:

I was going to make a final question but don't think there is any answer – how one copes with childlessness. I feel it is my problem – as my husband has pointed out – there's nothing wrong with him. He's even threatened divorce.

AID has given me some hope that I'll have a baby one day but I'm sure my husband isn't 100% for AID. Every so often he makes a remark like 'It's up to you to get pregnant – it's nothing to do with me now.' I know he feels a 'failure' and 'different' from other men and it's affecting our marriage. He also gets depressed sometimes and won't 'try' to get me pregnant by making love at the time of ovulation.

The second man is an only son, and very aware that he is not able to give his parents the grandchildren they want. Sometimes there are added problems when the husband comes from a culture where infertility is regarded as a woman's problem:

I got an appointment to attend my local hospital where they asked my husband to return after a few weeks with a semen sample. Unfortunately this caused more problems than I ever imagined. My husband just would not return with a specimen to the hospital, and when I myself returned to the hospital the doctor completely washed his hands of me saying he wasn't going to give me any fertility tests without checking my husband first.

Two years later the problem is still the same. Neither the husband nor the hospital has moved position. Yet the woman states that her husband adores children. What is the solution? This, at present, is a very little explored area, but one which urgently needs looking at.

Serious depression may be common amongst the involuntary childless: 'I, like lots of others, was treated by a consultant for my infertility, and my local GP for my depression and mild anorexia.' In a very few cases a woman feels suicidal:

At times I feel so sad for my husband because I keep telling him to divorce me and marry a woman who could give him children. It's all my fault we cannot have children. I really must make his life a misery, and yet I would rather die than for him to leave me. I really feel at the end of my tether at the moment. I even consider suicide, so my husband would be free to marry someone else and at least one of us would be happy.

Yet despite all the difficulties and the lack of success, some couples are determined to persevere against all possible odds.

I will not accept the fact that we will be childless. I have never had an abortion or miscarriage. I have heard of people conceiving with one ovary, one tube etc.

I am too strong-willed not to have another baby. As one doctor said: I make him smile. I always come back smiling and saying what do I know. He also said you are like a boxer and don't stay down on the ground for long.

She is *determined* to get somebody to look after whichever way possible and wants to prove that she can do it despite fostering rejections.

Even those who realise that they will never conceive find it difficult to break out of the circle of trying for a child:

What I would like is some help in accepting the state of childlessness, if that is the way ultimately it has to be. I thought I would get more used to the idea as the years went by and find other compensations, but it seems to remain an obsession with me.

We would like to contact members in our area who have the same sort of problems as us, so that we do not feel so isolated and abnormal. We realise that we are more fortunate than many, having two adopted children, but the same old feelings of desperation and sadness still occur.

A woman who eventually gave birth summarises the very subtle complexities and contradictions of life with and without children.

Now that I can look back on those childless years I am surprised at the intensity of my longing for a baby. I felt I was letting my mother down as she had been so upset when I married an Austrian and went to live abroad and I knew she would simply love a grandchild. Otherwise there were no pressures. In retrospect I am sorry I didn't enjoy the time we were just a couple even more. We did go out a lot and often went to Italy for the weekend or Zurich or Munich, all of which are near here. But we could have done more, and most of all I should have appreciated just being a pair more. Having no children brought us very close but I was often unhappy, which was so unnecessary as I had a very full and interesting life. I also tended to destroy relationships because of my jealousy if others had children.

The baby is wonderful and we are both so proud. However, I was amazed how difficult I found it is to adapt at first to being at home looking after the baby. I can only advise others to try to enjoy life today and not to think if it were otherwise it would be so much better. There are so many good things if we only appreciate them, but I know I am forgetting those strong feelings, the inborn need of women to have babies. A solution for the childless is certainly to channel those feelings in another direction if only a satisfactory way can be found – there lies the difficulty.

'If only…' says the woman with the child. 'If only…' says the woman without one.

Getting off the treadmill

There are two main ways in which a childless person may step off the ever-turning treadmill of infertility treatments and the search for a child. The first way is by bearing or acquiring a child. The second is by coming to terms with infertility and seeking another yardstick by which to measure the success of one's life. The childless, in general, do not have a great deal of choice as to which of the two ways is open to them.

Some very fortunate people achieve their own child. A couple who have waited $9^1/_2$ years write: 'It's a boy – Keith – born 23/1/82. 7lb 11oz and perfect! Labour only 2 hours!

Another couple had to wait even longer:

After 16 years of marriage our dream has finally come true.

Elaine and Stephen
announcing the birth of their son
James William
born
July 11th 1982
Weight 2lb 8$^1/_2$oz.
Sept 2nd 5lb 9oz.
Baby now at home.

Adoption, too, can bring great joy:

> Jenny gives us a lot of happiness and the sun shines in our home since she has joined us...

> She has turned our lives upside down and won our hearts completely, we love her so very very much. She is a very happy and contented baby and the joy she has brought us already is indescribable.

Fostering can bring great delight to those who have the personality and talents to undertake it successfully:

> Our family has grown quite suddenly. Whilst the eldest (14) is likely to move on in the near future, the other 3 (8,3 and 3 months) look like becoming permanent members of the family. We are obviously delighted at the prospect.

Donor insemination is the only way open to many, and it sometimes succeeds against all expectations:

> When our little boy was born, I realised that for me he was more special than I had imagined any child could ever be. All the doubts I'd ever had about him being the stranger were non-existent. He commanded all our love in his own right. Where he came from didn't matter one jot. My husband had my child, which he'd always wanted. As for our daughter, I knew long before she was born how extra specially marvellous she would be. Our son is so like his father, and our little girl is just like me, and they are both very much alike.

For one brave couple the bureaucratic hassles of overseas adoption pale into insignificance when their child arrives from Thailand.

> It took us 18 months to arrange for a child to be placed with us, but now we have a little boy who more than makes up for all the waiting. He was nearly 2 when we received him and we don't think it matters at all that he isn't a baby. The important thing is that he is here NOW!

What about the many who will neither be able to give birth, nor foster or adopt? Are they condemned to the treadmill for the rest of their lives? In one sense they cannot be, because they will eventually reach an age when none of their contemporaries is able to produce children either. But unless they have come to terms with their own situation before that, they might as well still be on the treadmill, as mentally and emotionally they have never left it. The grief which was for the children they never had is now transformed into grief for the grandchildren they will never have.

It may seem strange to suggest that one can grieve for the loss of something or someone that never existed. It goes counter to the familiar adage that 'you can't miss what you never had'. But this old saying is too trite. It is also a totally inaccurate measure of what it is, or is not, possible for people to grieve over. A child born into a loveless home is very much aware in adult life that something vital has been missing from his or her experience. It is quite possible to grieve over many different kinds of lost opportunity. This grief is possible because humans continually make comparisons between their own circumstances, and those of others whom they consider to be more fortunate than themselves.

With the childless, the grief over the loss of the life they would have had if they had had their own child is very real. They have been bereaved of the only conception of the future that they had ever considered, of the opportunity to be a mother or father, of the right to love in a very special way, of the joys of holding one's own beautiful, tiny, baby in one's arms.

The difference between the grief of a childless person, and that of someone mourning the loss of a loved person who has died, is that in the case of the childless, the grief is unfocused. Yet if one looks at the more usual grieving experience, it may be seen that in many respects the grief of the childless is similar to that of the bereaved. Murray Parkes, who has studied the experience of bereavement in depth, describes seven common aspects of grief. In assessing their relevance to the situation of the childless, it must be borne in mind that the list of points below does *not* provide a sequence of possible events or stages. The list summarises the most common reactions to bereavement:

(i)   A process of realisation, i.e. the way in which the bereaved person moves from denial, or avoidance of recognition of the loss, towards acceptance.

(ii) An alarm reaction – anxiety, restlessness and the physiological accompaniments of fear.

(iii) An urge to search for and find the lost person in some form.

(iv) Anger and guilt, including outbursts directed against those who press the bereaved person towards premature acceptance of his loss.

(v)   Feelings of internal loss of self, or mutilation.

(vi) Identification phenomena – the adoption of traits, mannerisms, or symptoms of the lost person, with or without a sense of their presence within the self.

(vii) Pathological variants of grief, i.e. the reaction may be excessive and prolonged, or inhibited and inclined to emerge in distorted form.[1]

With the exception, perhaps, of the sixth reaction, it is possible to identify all the reactions in the responses of the childless to their situation of loss. It has been shown how some of the childless initially try to deny the reality of their infertility. Anger is often expressed against those who try to make the childless aware of the need to face their loss. With some the feeling of self-mutilation comes over strongly. The pathological variants of grief are illustrated in the cases of women who consider or attempt suicide. The alarm reaction, and the urge to find the 'lost' person are experienced in the frantic attempts to find a way to have a child. All the above are illustrated in some way in the quotations from letters sent to the NAC office, which have been given in this chapter, and in the two previous chapters. The grief of many of the childless is real and terrible.

But at some point the need to grieve for the child who will never be born has to give way to the need to face life anew. The advice given by a mother-in-law to her daughter-in-law (see page 66) contains much wisdom. Until her daughter-in-law finally gave up the idea that there might be a chance, she would never be happy. Change does not happen, it has to be brought about by the individuals concerned. Nor is it an immediate process – it can take a long time, from the first decision to think or act in a different way, to eventual release from mental pain. The process is both internal and external, both aspects working together and reinforcing each other.

What the involuntary childless need to accept, to understand and to do, will form major themes of the second part of this book. This first part has emphasised the *problems* of childlessness. It is now time to look towards possible *solutions*. Just as the grief of a wife for her dead husband, a son for his dead mother, pass with time, and are gently assuaged, so it is possible for the childless to turn away from their secret sorrow, and to begin to live in tune with new conceptions and new purposes in life.

PART TWO

Working towards a solution

9

Childlessness: the three negations

In this chapter, the aim is to try to define what it is that makes the prospect of a life without children so fearful, and what are the consequences of this fear of childlessness. The fears will be dealt with under the headings of three negations – thwarted love, peripherality and genetic death. The thwarting of the desire to give parental love is a personal consequence of childlessness. The feeling of being peripheral to the family as it is perceived to work in our society is a social consequence of not having children of one's own. Genetic death is a biological description of the consequence of being without an heir; and as with many scientific views about social issues, there are philosophical implications that have to be considered. It must be stated at the outset, however, that individuals who are childless will not necessarily perceive all three feelings of negation as relevant to their situation. One of the negations will perhaps seem more important than the others, for different people, or at different times. Also they may not necessarily be the most important experience in the life of a childless person. Nevertheless, the three negations are consequences of childlessness that exist in some measure for those who do not have children. It is necessary, therefore, to understand the negations and their consequences if one is to be able to come to terms with childlessness.

Thwarted love: the personal consequence

In order to understand this consequence of childlessness a definition of love is needed. 'Love' seems capable of many interpretations. In the present context what is meant is a deeply felt emotion involving fondness and warmth of affection for another person. Often, some kind of intimacy is involved, and in some circumstances a sexual attraction or sexual relationship is part of the definition. The feelings expressed towards the other person may involve, under some circumstances, a willingness to sacrifice one's life for this second person. In many religions, love is seen as the highest emotional experience available to humankind. The apostle Paul, in his first letter to the Corinthians, writes:

> Love is patient, love is kind. It does not envy, it does not boast, it is not proud. It is not rude, it is not self-seeking, it is not easily angered, it keeps no record of wrongs. Love does not delight in evil but rejoices in the truth. It always protects, always trusts, always hopes, always perseveres. Love never fails.[1]

Although hope and faith are important ideals in the Christian life, it is love that is the most important. And much of the organisation of our present society seeks to find ways in which that love can be legitimately expressed.

It would seem that there are four particular times or occasions in life when love acts as a necessary element in the achievement of the wholeness of man or woman:

(i)   When, as children, we receive the love given to us by our parents; and later return that love.

(ii)   When we find a binding relationship as (young) adults, usually with a member of the opposite sex, with whom we can express the sexual side of our nature.

(iii) When, as a parent, we give love to our children, and later to our grandchildren.

(iv)   When we express our love towards good friends who have stood by us over the years.

For the majority of the childless the love they received from their parents will have been their first experience of love. Such love is central to the success of the child's first encounters with the world. The consequences of that love remain throughout life. The child, and later the adult, know that the love given to them is sure, even when they offend the parent or find themselves in serious trouble. Parents, in organising their lives around the needs of their children, give each child a confidence that grows from the feeling that he or she is important and of consequence to another. Where parental love is successfully expressed, it would seem natural for the children, in their turn, to wish to become parents, and to want to give love to their own children in return.

In some cases, there is a failure of parental love. The child of unloving parents enters adulthood with a serious handicap. Experiencing the love given by a parent is so crucial to the child's later security in adulthood that its absence can have profoundly negative effects which may take years to overcome. Birth control does nowadays give those who are aware of their own inadequacies (and believe they would not be good parents as a result) the chance not to become parents, if they choose.

However, for most parents, the pleasure and happiness shown by their children are very rewarding experiences, and the children in turn enjoy being part of their parents' source of happiness. As the children grow older they come to show love for their parents, in return for the love given to them; and the mutual love and dependence exist in different ways at different stages throughout the lives of both generations. The knowledge that the parent/child relationship can last well beyond childhood provides a link to the future for the parents, and is another rewarding aspect of the experience of parenthood.

As a child reaches adulthood a new kind of centrally important relationship may develop. This is often the result, in our society, of much experimentation with relationships during adolescence. The result is that there is usually the development of a long-term loving relationship, generally with the opposite sex, which enables the two partners to have sexual intercourse, making it possible for them to have a child of their own. For many, this kind of love is particularly intense and important, as it enables the sexual act to be a vehicle for the expression of love, while at the same time it fulfils the human biological functions of mating, reproduction and parenting.

This second experience of love does not always remain constant, as the divorce statistics will confirm.[2] It is not a static relationship, but develops as the two individuals involved develop and change over time. Some adults do not wish to become involved in such a close, binding relationship. Others prefer to develop a love relationship with a member of the same sex. However, in general, the long-term loving relationship is regarded as the most important of the experiences of love, and unlike the parent-child and child-parent relationships, it is usually chosen freely. No one can choose their biological parents. However bad the parent-child relationship, the two 'partners' in the relationship are bound for life. Though one may disinherit or refuse to acknowledge the other, the relationship and roles cannot be denied. This is not the case with the marital or conjugal relationship. It exists as the result of the choices made by each partner.

In the majority of relationships, the second kind of love eventually leads on to the third kind – that of parental love for the child or children of the union. Here the parent invests his or her love in the nurture of the young, and in providing a secure and prosperous environment in which the child can develop and grow. It involves quite a major adjustment in the lives of the parents, and is seen as a complete reversal of the role experienced in the first type of love – that of a child being given love by his or her parents. The first relationship emphasized the receiving of love; and being the object of another's responsibility. As a partner, one gives love, and assumes responsibility for another. There is satisfaction in watching the children progress towards adulthood, and later in watching one's children become parents themselves. There is the possibility of becoming a grandparent, which means that love given to one's children has the potential for another form of expression in later life – that of a grandparent's love for a grandchild. To many this is a most precious relationship, leading to much joy in later life.

Not all would accept that the fourth type of love relationship is essentially an expression of love. But the feeling of good friends towards one another can involve the mutual sharing of love. Like the relationship between partners in a marriage or long-term union, there is an element of freedom contained in the relationship. One chooses one's friends, even though it may be difficult to understand how the relationship began, or what sustains it. Friends provide pleasure and give one membership of an informal support group. Good friends can be a source of comfort and solace in times of sorrow and trouble, and as one's children grow up and become more independent, friendships may become more central to one's experience.

The childless face difficulties in experiencing some of the love relationships which are normally taken for granted. They are deprived of the third relationship, which legitimises the giving of love from a parent to a child, and they are affected by the fourth type of relationship when their friends have children, and they themselves do not. The childless may also perceive their parents' sadness at not having grandchildren, and they themselves cannot expect to have grandchildren either. They can only look on and observe others who are expressing the love relationships which have been denied to them as childless people. There is no legitimate substitution for most of these roles. Adoption and long-term fostering are only available to a very fortunate few, and in relationships with children it will not be possible to express the intimacy and sense of possession that is a normal part of the parent-child relationship.

There are several consequences that follow from these losses. Childless couples may have to absorb a greater part of their partner's love. Such couples can become very absorbed by one another. The concentration of love may become a burden, because love is not by nature exclusive, and it needs to be shared among several people, not just one, and the legitimate opportunity for this sharing is usually provided by children. Children divert parents from too great a concentration on each other, and they provide a channel to the outside world for the parents, by exploring the various enthusiasms of the younger generation as they become teenagers and young adults. It can be a disadvantage for a couple to be thrown back on one another; the only legitimate relationship based on intense love that they can express is given too much weight.

Secondly, while friends are experiencing the birth and development of the parent-child relationship, the childless are not able to share in the experience by having their own children. This can create stress and tension in a friendship, and in some cases lead to the ending of the friendship. The childless are unable to share in their friends' new absorption in the minutiae of family life, and the friends are not sure how to include the childless in their new, exciting and demanding lifestyle. The interests which the childless used to share with those who are now parents may come to seem unimportant to the latter. Conversely, the childless may feel distressed or guilty because they cannot share their friends' joys in having children; and the former may have to develop new friendships based on experiences which their friends with children cannot share.

As the childless watch their friends of the same generation go through the hassles and satisfactions of parenthood they find that there is no socially acceptable alternative path to follow if one is without children. The only generally accepted alternative is adoption, which is no longer a really viable alternative.[3] The childless, like those with children, wish to *give* love, and to be needed, in the way that a parent is needed for the survival and development of his or her child. The involuntary childless are deprived of the chance to give deeply committed love for a child. Most others take such an experience for granted, and may be completely unaware of the terrible deprivation felt by the childless.

The childless find that there is no one who really wants the love they have to give. They cannot join in the parenting role of others, as this is not socially approved. In our present society, the role of parenthood is not shared or extended beyond the confines of the nuclear family. Even grandparents have limited rights in disagreeing with the decisions of parents. Parents may be especially afraid that a childless friend might wish to subsume their own role. The childless themselves know that they would not willingly let anyone else interfere if they were parents, and so they understand why they cannot intervene in anyone else's family arrangements. But they suffer intense feelings of rejection as a consequence and have to bottle up a passion that threatens to overflow from time to time. They react in many different ways to try to control and overcome this problem, but as was said earlier,[4] they may in consequence be regarded as too 'self-centred', 'house-proud' or 'neurotic' to be able to have children. What they do as compensation may be considered by others to be a demonstration of the inadequacies which make them unsuitable to be parents.

It is true that too much concentration on one thing as a substitution can be counterproductive. It is very risky to put all one's energies into some activity or relationship that cannot bear the consequent strains. Some initial attempts to release thwarted love may lead one to understand fairly rapidly that no one person or activity can absorb all the passion and intensity that would have gone into caring for a child. The feelings of being deprived of the opportunity to give love are exacerbated by the constant emphasis of the media on the 'ideal family'. The need to belong to a family is seen by most as crucial. The distress that can be caused by family breakdown, and the effects of disturbed family relationships are evident to most social workers and psychiatrists. The family seems to exist to absorb some of the need for people to give and receive love (and antagonism) in ways that could not be controlled if they were permitted outside the confines of the family.

Sometimes a childless person develops the insight to see what is happening to him or her. One woman who wrote to the NAC office saw clearly what the problem was, even though she could not, at the time, find any solution.

I can't go round to my sisters's anymore since she's had the baby. I'm not just jealous. It's not even that I am not glad for her, or happy to have a nephew myself. What I can't stand is when Phillip automatically goes to her, presents his need for comfort and she replies in kind, glad to help, to be needed even when it is irritating, as it obviously is some days. It's not that she tries to stop me responding to Phillip – she's actually glad of the help. It's not even that I don't love Phillip – I do. Too much I feel, if my sister really knew. After crying at home every time I came back, I've thought about it… Yes, I'm angry with God for blessing my sister with what we both wanted and not me, but I'm not sure I really believe in God anyway. So I've been thinking what is it? What am I not facing? Andrew Staite said, when he wrote to me, that often you couldn't face the real problem and let go at things easier to attack on the side. Was I doing that I thought? I've realised I was and it's been painful and sometimes I've hated you at NAC for making me think of this. Basically I'm afraid. I've got all this love, maternal love, just waiting to be wanted and used up in me – I don't think it will ever be wanted or used. What am I going to do with it? Is it going to become anger and bitterness, or unresolved and hidden because I daren't talk about it because people will think I'm stupid or awkward to have around. It's really hard to feel your role as a person is redundant at 30. WHO IS GOING TO USE MY LOVE – WHO NEEDS IT?

How this writer is able to find an answer to the question as to who needs her love will depend on many factors. It will help if she and her partner are emotionally in harmony with one another. Where each partner nurses their own grievance to the exclusion of the needs of the other, there may be the seeds of an incipient tragedy. One man who very much wanted children tried to hide his disappointment by concentrating on the needs expressed by his wife.

> I've just got my head down and got on with life. She's made all the fuss. I've tried to help her. It's not been easy, she wants our baby so bad. I'd do anything, pay anything for her to have it. Helping her keeps the problem off me. I wanted kids too. I keep feeling if I let it get on top of me, like she does, I'd have to leave her and go and live with someone else that'd give me kids. I love her so I don't, but I know I'd love kids as much so I keep my head down and hope.

Eventually the wife became pregnant, but had a miscarriage. The husband later left her, and moved in with a girl who became pregnant by him. The wife, despite her grief, realised that she had been partly responsible for the break-up of their marriage. 'I drove him away. I didn't want him as much as a baby'. Neither of them was able to articulate their secret feeling that they had each been thwarted of the opportunity to express parental love to a child.

Sometimes a couple may understand their mutual needs, and work together to try to solve the problem. But the solution is not always easy. One couple, who discovered early in their life together that they would not be able to have children, tried to work out a solution that would enable them to have contact with children. The wife decided to become a teacher, and eventually became a very successful remedial teacher. She was recommended to apply for the post of home/school liaison officer, but decided against this because she enjoyed teaching, and the opportunities it gave her for direct contact with children. She felt that she had more time than most of the other teachers to deal with the problems of children in distress, and that this was one of her most important functions. One day one of her pupils, from a very troubled home, ran away from home and came to her house for help. She gave the child hospitality and care, at the same time informing the parents and the appropriate authorities. She was pleased that the girl felt able to turn to her, but was worried when the parents said that she 'could have her'. The girl had to stay the night until the social services could sort out the problem the next day. The couple befriended the child's parents, and as a result befriended the girl, to her benefit, as far as anyone could tell. It took time, money and patience trying to help this troubled girl with a difficult family.

However, the Headmaster of the school called the teacher into his office one day, and said that he felt he must talk to her about this special relationship she had with the girl. Did she not think that the relationship was unprofessional, in view of her role as a teacher? Was she not going too far in this case, to compensate for her own childlessness? Although he felt that she worked well with disturbed children, and her own needs obviously provided the right, positive motivation for this work, he thought she had gone too far in the present case. The teacher and her husband both felt angry, and at the same time guilty. She felt her childlessness had caused her to be assumed to be unprofessional. What was the Headmaster's real point? Was it that she should not be involved with pupils outside school? Or was it that people with special personal needs to work with children should not become involved in tasks that required special skills in dealing with vulnerable children? Might the special personal needs interfere with their ability to exercise the special skills in the most objective and useful way? The woman consulted the social worker involved with the family, who felt that the family would not benefit from the couple's immediate withdrawal, but that withdrawal had to be planned in the long-term, in the interests of all parties. Ironically, it had been the social worker talking to the Headmaster about the need for a planned withdrawal of the couple from their work with the family that had resulted in the woman's most distressing interview with the Headmaster. It is difficult to know whether he was interpreting the social worker's suggestions in a different spirit from that in which they had been given. But even allowing for a possible misunderstanding in communications, the effect on the couple was still devastating. They lost confidence in their ability to deal with children and went through a long period of depression and reappraisal. Eventually the woman trained for social work, and she and her husband fostered two children.

It is very easy for those who are parents to condemn the childless for any attempt they make to compensate for the thwarting of their desire to love. It is easy to dismiss what they say, or misinterpret what they do on the grounds that 'they can't possibly know anything about it – they haven't got children.' It is comforting, when one has an argument with the teacher of one's children, to be able to say of her that 'she's really an old spinster, so she doesn't understand about children – it's just a job to her.' The only comfort for the childless is that children are often capable of making accurate judgments about who does and who does not understand them, and they may be quite realistic about their own parents' limitations. But, of course, children do not generally reveal this; otherwise, where would their next meal come from?

The childless, single or married, are not different to others in their desire to belong and to love. The difference is that there are very few legitimate outlets available to them to express these needs. Ultimately, most of the childless will reach some form of compromise. They will learn to restrain their feelings, and they will find alternative compensations. But it may be a slow, sometimes painful, learning process in the meantime. Much will depend on the support they are given by friends, relatives and colleagues.

Peripherality: the social consequence

In the previous section the experience of thwarted love was seen as a very personal loss, a negation of one of the strongest human needs. To be an integrated, secure individual one must be able to give, as well as receive, love. Peripherality, though it has an impact on the lives of the individuals who experience it, is essentially a social consequence of childlessness.

The family is still considered by many to be the basic unit of society. There is an assumption that the family by its very existence and history implies ties, duties and dependencies.[5] When the nature of the roles one might expect to find in the family undergoes some kind of change, it requires an adjustment of previous social perceptions of the family. The conventional primary roles of greatest importance in the drama of the family are those of child, spouse, parent and grandparent. [6] There are also secondary roles of lesser importance – cousin, aunt or uncle, brother or sister, great aunt or uncle. Family roles revolve around the events experienced by these networks of people to whom one has some kind of blood relationship, the primary roles being generally of most significance, and having the greatest potential for satisfaction or sorrow. Even where families are seen to split up, or key members to opt out of their assigned roles, or new families are created from units of previous families, and the family itself is seen to be undergoing radical changes, the concept of family still seems to hold good for a variety of social, economic and political reasons.[7]

In previous generations there was little choice as to which roles one played in the family, particularly for women. Today it is possible to avoid parenthood and consequent grandparenthood if one makes certain choices and decisions. However, most of the other family roles still demand some kind of duty or tie, unless one lives too far away from the family for the ties to be meaningful, or one is too estranged from relatives for the roles to be still valid. There are, however, times in life when the primary roles are less important or less demanding than at other times. One period is adolescence and young adulthood, when there is a greater need to relate to friends and peer groups in order to find a partner with whom to share later adult life. This stage may be long or short, depending on the individual, but it is a stage between the role of child and that of spouse or partner for many people. Later in life when one's children are leaving home, and no grandchildren have yet been born, there is a time when the parental role is coming to an end and a second 'between' stage may come about. Again, this period can be long or short, depending on when one's children become parents themselves. Finally, often after the death of one's partner, there is the experience, perhaps solitary, of old age. Although one may be a grandparent, it does not necessarily mean that one has more than occasional contact with one's children. For many old people, life is not centred around the family, even if the elderly person would like it to be.

These periods in life when the primary family roles are not so demanding are times when the lives of childless people do not seem to be very much out of step with the lives of their peers. In some cases, the childless may be said to be better prepared for times of living alone than are their peers who have had families. Such times demand self-motivation and an ability to enjoy things for what they are; they are not times when there are satisfactions to be derived mainly from family life. Sometimes the childless can be of comfort to others in these periods. One parent wrote:

I often think childless couples miss seeing the good side of things going for them. My children have left me, and I felt high and dry on a beach with nowhere to go. It was my neighbour, who had never had children, who quietly chivvied me into doing new things. It was only then I realised she was the best friend I ever had and stopped feeling sorry for her.

Another woman wrote:

My mother was a pain in the neck when we left home. She couldn't let us go. We were everything. There was never anything else really important in her life. Well I'm not going to make that mistake. It's the one positive thing about childlessness – you learn that other things in life than children and family can be enjoyed.

Although there are times when the childless can act as a source of inspiration to those who have had children, and although there are people who do not gain great satisfaction from their parental role, there are some serious consequences in not being a parent. One has only to measure the importance of the times when parents are not fully occupied with family life, against the times when children dominate their interests, and are absolutely central to the meaning of family life. It becomes evident that, in relation to the family, the childless will take on a secondary role, on the periphery. They may be aunts or uncles, but they will not have a central role in the family. This raises questions of 'belonging'. To whom do the childless 'belong', or who 'belongs' to them? 'I am one of those people who define in other people's eyes how lucky others are to have children. We have no close relatives, no-one belongs to us.'

This woman's friends measure themselves against what she appears to lack – a sense of belonging. Although she has her good and bad days, like everyone else she feels that she needs her friends more than they seem to need her. She thinks they secretly feel sorry for her: 'They think I don't know what I'm missing. They think I'm too lonely. They see me as someone in a way to look after because I have no-one else.' Many childless couples experience this sort of response from friends and relatives. Yet these people often fail to realise that the childless make judgments in return. By allowing themselves to be helped, the childless may feel that they are enabling others to feel useful: 'They need me but I see they do not know they do. I let them feel I need them more – I do need them and by using them I have a purpose. I can give in return.'

At first sight, peripherality may not seem too serious a negation. Not all families are close, not all parents find deep satisfaction in attempting to fulfil their destined role. The distancing of the childless from friends who have children takes place slowly, and it may not be immediately apparent that a rift is being formed. But it is very hard to share the interests of those who are absorbed by their children, when one does not share the same absorption. And as time goes by a childless couple may be the only survivors of a group of friends or relatives who are now fully occupied in bringing up a family. It is not always easy to find new people with whom to replace the friendships of the past. If one joins a group, it is likely that the majority of the members will belong to the age groups that are not typically involved with family affairs; they are probably much younger or older than oneself. This is not a reason to despise these different groups of people, but it may be hard to find a common ground on which to form a closer relationship. Parents, because of the demands of their children, often make friends with other parents who have children of a similar age; it helps to lessen the burden by spreading child-care responsibilities, and enables each of the adults involved to snatch a well-earned period of rest, enjoyment and companionship, possibly on some kind of informal rota basis. Where a childless couple have maintained a close relationship with friends who have children, the childless couple may become involved in family activities and outings that are enjoyed by all, but the relationship with the children, indeed with the whole family, may still be peripheral. The childless may find that the enjoyment experienced during the occasional contact with children acts to strengthen their feelings of isolation when they are on their own again:

Although we have adjusted emotionally, we are finding considerable problems socially. Our main problem is that the fact that we do not have children tends to isolate us from couples who do have a family.

Public holidays can be particularly painful for the childless. Very few of their friends are available, as they are mostly involved in family activities. One can wander round parks and zoos on bank holidays, and watch families bored to tears by each other, or falling out with each other. But the important thing is that they are bored or falling out *together*. They are fulfilling their function as family units. No one requires that they be happy fulfilling these functions; there is just some deeply felt and shared sense that they are doing the right thing in acting as a family.

Because large numbers of the childless have partners, it is easy for others to misunderstand their situation. The childless have comfort and friendship from each other, but they are often denied the rewards that come from being involved with children. People may not realise the extent of a childless couple's aloneness, or loneliness:

I am now forty. I was an only child. My parents, aunts and uncles are dead. My husband's family live far away, we have little contact. To all intents and purposes we have no relatives only each other. That is something, of course, but no-one has any duty to us, any obligation. We can count on no-one other than ourselves.

I took my friends' children to the zoo. We had a lovely day, full of fun. I enjoyed it all. I went round the zoo pointing it all out to them – no-one thought it odd. Three days before my husband and I went just to see it before we took them. It was a totally different experience. Surrounded by families and their enthusiastic children we wandered alone like strangers among the herd.

The effects of peripherality thus cause the childless to feel cut off, left out, or like 'strangers among the herd'. As one gets older, the tendency is for one to become more solitary, and to find that one is to be solitary from an early age in life can be hard to bear. Despite the many shortcomings of the modern family, it does provide a means to 'belong'; and to feel that one belongs to no one can be very frightening.

On reflection it seems a little strange that the concept of 'the family' is regarded as so sacrosanct, when in reality so many people are 'excluded' from it, or made peripheral through no fault of their own. It seems ironic that the childless feel so strongly about their exclusion from an institution which in general has not treated them particularly well; and because of the way it functions at present, leaves them with a very minor role to play. For their own peace of mind, it might be easier if they thought less of family, and more of alternative ways to be accepted as members of a differently perceived society. But it has to be understood that peripherality is the experience of those who stand on the edge of the society they wish to join. The majority of the childless ask nothing more than to be ordinary, unexceptional members of the family-based society that so many people with children take for granted. Peripherality leaves them with an absence of role within the family; a sense of not belonging, and of being of little importance in the family; a need to search for alternatives that are not typical for their generation; and a struggle to discover what their life can mean if they are to have no part in rearing a new generation.

Genetic death: the genetic and philosophical consequence

The third negation experienced by the childless is called 'genetic death'. It is somewhat more complex in conception than thwarted love and peripherality. It deals with the difficult question of the roles available to people who are not contributing genetically to the future of humankind. Genetic death is the situation where a person contributes no genes to the future genetic pool of the human population. It is not an easy topic to discuss, as a full understanding of its meaning and importance would involve a detailed study of genetics, philosophy and many other related subjects. We have attempted here to set out some very general ideas, which may later need to be refined and reworked. It would not be appropriate to develop these ideas within the framework of the present book, but it is hoped to develop them, in a different context, some time in the future.

Genetically speaking, as far as the biological future of the human race is concerned, a childless person is a dead end. This is something which people find hard to accept, or to discuss. Some childless people are not concerned about this at all. There is a feeling that men are concerned more about it than women. In large families the help of unmarried or childless aunts and uncles may still be utilised to ensure the successful nurture of children, just as the survival and reproductive success of bees is secured by the nurturing of brother and sister bees, not of the parent. But relatives of secondary role importance are not needed to ensure the successful future of the offspring in the typical, small, western family.

At a different, more philosophical level, genetic death is also important, because in some ill-defined way the nurture of children aids an individual's personal growth, and helps him or her maintain personal continuity in the human experience. Peripherality and thwarted love are in a way a consequence of genetic death. It is that death which excludes the childless from the mainstream of the human experience. Is there a role for a genetic dead end? It is a problem for many people, and is expressed in different ways:

> I look at the people who have children, some of whom are terrible people and I think they'll be part of the future and I won't.

> Look at all these people who don't want kids and have them – just like that. Why are they going to be in the future and not me who wants them very much and can't?

These two quotations from letters show an element of bitterness, but they are influenced by a fear of a loss of any stake in the future. The following letter expresses this in a different way:

> My sister said whats it matter you won't have children. You can share mine. This is not really true because I can't share them as their mum but I know she meant well. The truth is though, isn't it, that if I am never the main influence on a child through to when it leaves home and have never had a baby I'm just a backwater. Someone to be remembered now and again and be kind to at Christmas. I wanted to be part of the next generation not the last of the Mohicans.

Men describe the same experience with a slightly different emphasis. They may have the feeling that they have failed in their responsibility towards a whole line of ancestors, or they may fear loss of social status:

> Who will carry on the family name? I'm the last. All my ancestors are made nothing by my sterility.

> You tell me it's not the end of the world not having children. No – but it's the end of my bit in the world isn't it?

> In our valley family is everything. Not being a father is to lose face. You don't matter really see, because there's no-one looking out for you.

> I'm a dead man really now. Why not wrap it all up I say before I have to rely on strangers? I never thought I would come to this, dead before my time.

That it might be painful to lose a biological stake in the next generation may not occur to many people. This sense of loss seems to reflect some kind of underlying fear. A fear of being forced to depend upon strangers, a fear of being isolated in times of trouble, with no one to help fight one's battles with the world.

The childless may also suffer from another more subtle kind of loss. This is expressed in the following excerpt from a letter written by a woman who was herself a parent. "'Well, you've no kids, you can do as you like". I think that's a pity, because you are making little things most people do in passing much more important than they are.' This letter was written to NAC in response to a newspaper article which explained how childless couples had to take up new interests to help them overcome their grief. The woman suggests that it is a pity that the childless will be denied the rewards of the experience which she herself has had, but at the same time she manages to imply that any alternative which the childless might consider must be trivial, in comparison with the experience of raising a family. That this is manifestly untrue, when one looks at the achievements throughout history of those who have not had children, does not occur to her. But her attitude does reflect a fear expressed by many of the childless – a fear that nothing they can do will be of any real or lasting value.

The above responses to the fear of genetic death are primarily social responses. They are about fears of being pitied or downgraded in the social groups within which the childless seek to establish their social identity. But in the long term it cannot be particularly important whether one's genes are or are not part of the future gene pool. It matters in the short life of an individual, but in the human story, over many, many generations, it cannot be of much importance.

Genetics is the study of heredity. Its prime interest is in which 'genes' are passed on from generation to generation, and in what causes some gene successions to be more successful than others. In reproduction, one half of the genes of each individual are shared with those of the partner, through the union of egg and sperm to create new life. The act of conception is, however, not the whole story. The young must be nurtured to a greater or lesser degree, to ensure their survival. Successful reproduction involves both successful fertilisation and the parental investment of time and care to ensure that the fertilised egg reaches adulthood. Both the urge to achieve copulation, and the urge to nurture young, seem to be strong in mammalian species like man, where it takes a long time for an infant to reach maturity and to be able to look after itself.

In some species, less time and parental investment is involved, but in these cases much larger numbers of fertilised young are produced, to ensure the survival of a few. The genetic story of a species is about ensuring its future through reproduction. Unsuccessful reproducers have no part in that future, except during their own limited lives. In many mammalian species, for example, dominant males prevent the copulation of females with other males, to ensure the survival of only the strongest or most cunning animals of the species.

Does this process of reproduction and nurturing for successful survival have anything to suggest for the reproductively unsuccessful? To answer this question it is important to stress that there are two essential components to successful reproduction, as mentioned above. Firstly, there must be successful fertilization and birth; secondly, the young must be nurtured until adulthood. With regard to the human species, as suggested on page 91, there has until recently been a role for the childless in helping to nurture the young in the traditional larger family, where the parents had to disperse their care over large numbers of offspring. Adoption and fostering were also at one time available to many of the childless, to enable them to adopt a nurturing role in the successful rearing of children who were later to become parents themselves, thus taking part in the successful reproduction of the next generation of the human species. The general absence, in the present day, of traditional nurturing roles of this kind has led many of the childless to seek representation in the human future by pursuing medical fertility treatments. Some have also sought other forms of nurture, taking on social roles in some way connected with the nurture of the next generation, in areas such as teaching, social work, and many kinds of voluntary work; and others have expressed their need to nurture through taking part in the care of animals. But for the majority of the childless the future is now, for a variety of reasons, seen to be secured through access to new medical techniques and expertise.[8]

It is difficult to know whether the change in emphasis of the solutions sought by the childless is due, at a very fundamental level, to the unavailability of nurturing roles. There has never been a time in the past when reproductive success could be secured through medical intervention on any measureable scale, as is possible today. It might be possible to carry out research, by interviewing those who adopted a child at some earlier point in the present century, to ascertain whether they would have preferred to give birth to their own child if this had been possible. But it would not reveal anything about human preferences in general. The stigma attached to illegitimacy, which is still a disadvantage in many ways in many societies, suggests that reproduction is only desirable under certain socially determined conditions.[9] It is not regarded as the solution to a man or woman's needs for representation in the genetic pool of the future, if the fertilization takes place outside the confines of what a society regards as legitimate or correct. (A certain old lady, known to the writers of this book, has had to be persuaded, on more than one occasion, that royalty does *not* have blue blood; and that the heir to the throne is not polluting the royal line by marrying and reproducing outside the 'Royal' Family).

In many countries of the West, however, relaxations of traditional ideas about the circumstances under which reproduction is permitted have helped to make it easier for greater numbers of the childless to seek medical treatment. Yet there are still problems not so easily soluble. Fertilisation requires a genetic contribution from two people, and it is often forgotten that in many reproductively unsuccessful partnerships only one of the partners is likely to be infertile. This raises difficult questions for the fertile partner as to whether to remain committed to the partnership. In some societies, irrespective of which partner is infertile, the man has grounds for divorcing the woman.[10] Although this may seem an injustice, it is genetically an efficient selection process, as it enables other possibilities for reproduction, through different combinations of partners; and it increases the odds that a partnership will lead to fertilisation.

Many of the new reproductive techniques enable a couple to be successful without having to resort to divorce or to look for a new partner. What may often be needed for successful reproduction is some kind of third-party involvement. This is the case with artificial insemination by donor, and with surrogate mothering. Egg donation, where a woman receives the egg of another women through in-vitro fertilisation is another, very recent, technique.[11]

There are many moral questions raised about the use of these advanced reproductive techniques, but they do at least make it possible for a potentially fertile partner in a childless relationship to succeed reproductively. Yet there may be some genetic doubt about helping the infertile partner to reproduce, since it could be said in some cases that some kind of genetic selection had already taken place to bring one reproductive line to an end. There is, however, medical evidence to suggest that much infertility simply involves malfunctions in the reproductive system.[12] It could also be claimed that the ability to manipulate reproduction is itself a genetic advance.

The discovery of new technologies that help reproduction has freed many otherwise infertile people from total dependence on chance.[12] This is a very new phenomenon, and needs some examination. Reproduction has always been a rather blind and chancy affair, totally dependent on the successful transmission of genes. If genes could not be transmitted, that was the end. The new technology, however, suggests that we will not now have to remain so dependent upon chance. New possibilities are at once opened up, not only for the childless, but for humanity in general. It becomes possible to contemplate genetic selection to 'improve' the human race, with all that is involved in making decisions as to what an 'improvement' is. The new technologies challenge dependence on chance.

But where did that challenge originate? In effect, the challenge originated in the minds of researchers and medical practitioners who were anxious to understand and enhance reproduction. The ideas they had, and the technologies they developed to give them effect, were, in an indirect way, making them 'parents' of the children subsequently born. This is a very important development, since, in the past, children were solely the result of genetic succession. In some ways those who have pioneered new reproductive techniques can be said to be like 'marriage brokers' who, in bringing a young couple together, are helping to arrange a new gene succession.

The challenge to chance, in making possible certain gene successions, is only one aspect of the development of human abilities to control and change the world which we inhabit. The new reproductive techniques are also the products of talented minds, looking with critical insight into the nature of what is regarded as known, showing that what has come to be accepted as unchangeable, is, in fact, open to change. Of all the animal species that inhabit the world, humans alone seem to be capable of transforming the conditions of that world to their own advantage. What was once attributed to the will of the gods or spirits is now seen to be under control of man and woman.

It is important for the childless that they should understand this, for many more things than just reproduction are thereby validated, in terms of their contribution to the human future. Ideas are also transmitted, and modified from one generation to another. Written records, customs handed down over the centuries, art, poetry, music, religion, all contribute to the pool of human experience and remain part of one's cultural heritage, to be passed on to future generations. One does not have to be a scientist or artistic genius in order to become part of the future. People contribute to the future by contributing to the age and society within which they live. It may be hard for the childless to appreciate this, but posterity may not judge in the same way as one's peers do, and after one's death one will be remembered for what one did and for what one was as a person, as much as for the descendants one produced.

Nevertheless, for those for whom genetic death is perceived as a powerful negation of one's role and influence in life, comfort may be difficult to accept. Like thwarted love and peripherality, it defines the condition of the childless in relation to themselves, their society and the future. The three negations dealt with in this chapter are not special to the childless; they may be experienced by others under different circumstances. Conversely, some of the childless may not be particularly affected by the important negations. But for those who are attempting to come to terms with childlessness, and to readjust to a different view of the future, it may be helpful to face the fears underlying their sense of loss. When a fear is faced and understood, its power to harm may slowly begin to diminish.

10

Adoption

A close reading of the first part of this book may have led the reader to question whether adoption is any longer a viable solution to the problem of childlessness. The statistics will have shown how few babies are available for adoption.[1] As a result, it has become very difficult for young couples to be accepted as adoptive parents, and virtually impossible for older childless couples. The adoption vetting process has become more and more stringent as social services departments and adoption agencies try to ensure that the very few babies available go to the best homes. For all practical purposes, adoption is only a possible solution for a very limited number of the childless.

Yet adoption does need to be considered as a possible solution to childlessness. It is still seen as a solution by both the childless and those with whom they come into contact, both professionally and informally. Adoption is frequently recommended to people undergoing fertility tests and investigations. Sometimes a doctor or consultant will suggest that a couple would be wise to apply, if there are any doubts about the likely outcome of treatment. Friends will often tell a couple not to wait for the results of tests or treatment, but to begin the process of adopting right away. Parents may suggest it, if they feel that the misery of a couple undergoing treatment is too great. Many couples worried about infertility will decide to apply for adoption, irrespective of who suggests it to them. It seems the natural thing to do. Most people know of families with adopted children. Many people hear stories to the effect that a couple had their own natural children after adopting, and thus some see adoption as an aid to the treatment of their own infertility. There is no evidence to establish that myth.[2] People do have their own children after adoption, but at no greater rate than do people of their age who do not adopt. Irrespective of the reality, it is part of our folk wisdom that adoption exists to help those who wish to found or extend their family.

The decision to try to adopt may mark the first stage of acceptance by a couple that they may not be able to have their own child. This involves a recognition that the role of genitor (natural parent) may have to be regarded as lost, and that the role of nurturer should be pursued. There will not be the same relationship with an adopted child as there would be with a natural child. Any sense of a relationship with the embryo and foetus during pregnancy will be denied to the adoptive mother. The adoptive parents will miss the experience of birth, and the opportunity for the development of a relationship with the baby over the first few weeks, months or years of its life. These early stages are full of excitement and possibilities for many natural parents. In later life, too, the adoptive, nurturing parents will become very aware that they are not the child's natural parents. They have an obligation to explain this to the child at some point. Once this is known to the child, however he or she takes it, for good or ill, the admission has been made and the truth recognised. People think of adoption as a replacement for a natural child. It is actually a substitution, an alternative that enables one to offer one's services as a parent. In earlier times this did not really matter, as there were more children in need of being adopted than there were people willing to adopt. It matters now, because the selection process is likely to eliminate many people, and a couple do need to understand that adoption does not mean merely obtaining a family by another means. A social worker will expect a couple to understand that, and to realise why the selection process has to be so rigorous and selective. The social worker, in turn, needs to understand that, for the childless, the act of applying for adoption is a recognition that they are infertile or childless, even if they are unable to admit this openly.

The odds are heavily against any couple who apply for adoption. Only about one in ten is likely to get on to a list for investigation.[3] This does not mean that a large number are rejected as a result of the selection process. Very few are rejected if they are fully vetted. Some couples never complete the process, others find that even when it is complete there are still no babies or young children available. There are no reliable estimates of the number of childless couples wanting to adopt. No statistics of enquiries about adoption are kept, as most lists of potential adopters are closed. The National Association for the Childless believe that about a third of its members are trying to join an adoption list. If this is translated into numbers nationally, it suggests that about 250,000 couples will be currently trying to become adoptive parents.[4]

However, some childless people do successfully complete the adoption process and receive an adoptive child of their own. Some successfully foster a child or group of children. For those who decide it would be right for them to adopt or foster, this chapter tries to put the experience into some kind of meaningful perspective. Adoption is such a fraught, distressing and uncertain process, that it is very important for vulnerable groups such as the childless to understand fully the nature of the course on which they are embarking.

It must be accepted at the outset that because so few babies and very young children are available for adoption, even those who would make excellent parents, and are accepted by an agency as potential adopters, may never receive a child. It is very much a 'numbers game' and must depend to a certain extent on luck. Another thing that needs to be understood is that adoption or any other form of childcare is by law primarily selected in the best interests of the child. The adoption authority is seeking a satisfactory home or placement for the child. It is not in the business of fulfilling the needs of the childless. And in the current political and social climate the needs of the childless are sometimes viewed with suspicion.

The background to current approaches and attitudes to childcare policy is provided by the 1975 Children Act, which enables certain children and babies to be freed for adoption without necessarily waiting for parental permission. Though the Act was formulated to enable children in care to achieve some kind of permanency in their home and family life, to avoid the deleterious effects of long-term insecurity in childhood, it has been interpreted by some groups in society as a means by which the poorer and more deprived social groups are 'robbed' of their children because they are unable to provide the same standard of care for them as the more affluent can.[5] Likewise, children of other races, who were once considered 'hard to place', because white parents preferred to adopt white children, are now recognised as being in need of parents of their own race. Transracial adoption is regarded by many as inadequate, as it is thought that white parents will not be able to bring up a child of another race to feel proud of his or her racial identity, or to help the child cope with the racism he or she could well be exposed to as an adult. At its strongest this view is expressed in statements regarding transracial adoption as a form of 'genocide' by depriving races of their children.[6] Likewise, the thinking behind current approaches to inter-country adoption reflects similar views about the desirability of children being brought up within their own culture.[7]

This very negative background has been given so that those who decide they should try to adopt are aware that what they are doing may not necessarily be regarded as an altruistic act in the interests of society. Nevertheless, it is recognised that there are many successful adoptions of all kinds of children, and many adopted children grow up into secure, loving adults who bring great happiness to their families.[8]

In deciding what kind of adoption or fostering to apply for, certain factors need to be kept in mind. For healthy babies, most adoption agencies have an upper age limit for would-be adopters, which may be as low as 33 for the woman in some cases.[9] Thus adoption of healthy (white) babies is virtually restricted to the younger age groups of the childless. There are generally fewer age restrictions for the adoption of children with special needs – older children and teenagers, groups of brothers and sisters, children with physical or mental handicaps.[10] Here it is more important that the adoptive parents have the special qualities needed to cope with the extra physical or emotional needs of the children. So this is likely to be a type of adoption that can only appeal to those childless people who feel they have the ability to do it.

For the older childless who have the means to do so, inter-country adoption is at present probably the only way they will be able to find a baby or very young child to adopt. It is a risky and expensive process, fraught with hazards and bureaucratic complications. At present it operates in a fairly ad hoc fashion, but the British Agencies for Adoption and Fostering (BAAF) are anxious to introduce some type of regulation to control the practice of inter-country adoption, to ensure that the children involved are genuine orphans without any kind of family support, and to make sure that those who adopt the children in this country are judged to be capable of giving each child the appropriate form of care.[11] Transracial adoption of a child living in this country is possible under certain circumstances, but this, like inter-country adoption, is probably only appropriate for a limited number of the childless.[12]

Fostering, which is another possible way for the childless to enjoy family life, should not be confused with adoption. With adoption, a child legally belongs to his or her adoptive parents. Fostering is 'looking after someone else's child in your home as if it were your own'.[13] The assumption is generally that the child will return to the parental home at some point in the future. There are different types of fostering, short term and long term, and after a period of five years or more foster parents may apply to adopt a child. This does not mean that adoption will be granted, though it is more likely with long-term fostering of an older child. But it is stressed by the adoption agencies that fostering is not the back door to adoption, and that foster parents have to get used to seeing a child they have come to love leaving their home.[14] NAC received the following letter from two members:

Dear Sir,

We are emigrating to _____ in six weeks time, so wondered if you could cancel our *Nack*. Also we wanted to thank you for all the interesting and helpful articles we have read in *Nack*.

After nine years of childlessness, we now have resigned ourselves to the fact that we will not have children of our own, which we still yearn for. We have in fact been fostering for a year and at the moment have a lovely baby girl 'Kirsty' who was one two days ago, we have had her nine months and have tried to adopt her but to no avail, one reason was that we weren't on their list, although she was only meant to be with us six weeks, she is now going for adoption to someone else, which will break our hearts, but we know she will be dearly loved by her new parents, which is little comfort really, because now she is part of us and she knows us as Mummy and Daddy. We think its unfair on her too, as she has always been very insecure and it took us months to win her confidence so now she is settled down beautifully. She now has to be moved again. We have even spoken to the director of social services, but apparently they must keep to the book and cannot make any exceptions to the rules which makes us, friends and family very angry, even our friends have protested to the authorities, to say Kirsty should stay with us. But we have been told 'no' in no uncertain terms, we can't have her, so we have decided to emigrate and start a new life and perhaps adopt in _____ although it isn't easy to adopt a baby there also. Well, carry on your good work and I hope a lot more people will join in the future and have more luck than us and eventually have a baby.

Thanks again.

Mr. & Mrs. _____

The rights and wrongs of this case apart, loss of their beloved foster-child is a devastating experience for this couple, and one can only hope that they find some happiness in their new life. Again it has to be said that it seems likely that fostering will be suitable for relatively small numbers of the childless.

Once the decision to apply has been made, what should be expected? The initial difficulty may be in finding a social services department or adoption agency willing to accept the couple on their list of applicants for consideration:

We've been to fourteen adoption agencies and our local authority – all the lists are closed. What do they do – say try someone else. What do we do when we run out of those someone else's?

It's been five years since we tried to get on a list for adoption. No one yet has even agreed to consider our application and then tell us to try others we've already tried whose lists are closed.

We are luckier than most, we have been accepted by an adoption agency and are waiting for a baby to be referred. However, our social workers have always pointed out that they may never have a child they can place with us, and we could run out of time. So in the meantime, we are continuing to try and be accepted by other agencies, such an enormously difficult task. Adoption societies' lists appear to be permanently closed and their standard reply is to suggest we try other agencies. WE HAVE! Why can't all agencies and social services departments work together?

The only advice here can be to persevere in the hope that somewhere, at some time, a couple will be lucky and find an agency or their local social services department willing to consider them. It does suggest, however, that a decision to apply for adoption needs to be taken long before a couple reach the age-limits stipulated by agencies, if they are to have any chance of success, however small.

Even if a couple are eventually accepted for consideration, it must be assumed that the enquiries will take a considerable time, lasting possibly over years. Sometimes this can lead to considerable frustration and disappointment. Here is one couple's experience:

Summary of progression of adoption application

1981

7 May   Wrote to County Council Social Services Department to enquire about adoption.

2 June   Preliminary interview with social worker – completed police and health authority forms, and told to expect contact in approximately one month.

19 August   Wrote to social worker to query why we had not heard from her – NO REPLY.

1 Oct.   Wrote again to social worker – NO REPLY.

1982

8 Jan.   Telephoned social worker, who asked me to ring again mid February: 'I will try to get something started then.'

16 Feb.   1. Telephoned social worker, who explained that she was too busy to deal with our adoption application and that waiting list was closed.
            2. Wrote to Client Care and Placement Section of Social Services at Central Office to enquire whether our case could be considered by another Adoption Advisor who had more time.

22 Feb.   Letter from Central Office, advising that my letter had been passed on to the Area Organiser.

4 April	Wrote again to Central Office, as we have not heard from Area Organiser.
14 April	Letter from Area Organiser asking us to confirm that we still wished to be considered: confirmation of this sent by return of post.
6 May	First visit by a new social worker.
July	Last visit by new social worker. Advised that we should be notified of panel's decision approximately one month after submission of her report, and completion of medical examinations – i.e. by end of October. New social worker announced that she was leaving the department as she was pregnant!
30 Nov.	Telephoned original social worker, who could not trace our papers and, therefore, assumed they were at Central Office. I was told that this part of the proceedings takes a long time!

1983

12 Feb.	Wrote to Client Care and Placement Section at Central Office to advise change of employment and try to establish cause of delay.
3 March	Letter received from Chairman of the Adoption Panel, explaining that the information given by second social worker was not accurate and advising that 'it appears most likely that a decision will be made within the next few weeks'.
8 June	Wrote to Area Organiser to query why we had not heard anything further – NO REPLY.
19 June	1. Telephoned Area Organiser – told to ring back and speak to the original social worker's clerk.
	2. Telephoned the clerk who said, 'I'll have a rummage and see whether I can come up with anything.'
	3. Clerk telephoned back to advise that we had been accepted by the panel during the latter part of March! Advice from Central Office had been marked for second social worker's attention and had not been dealt with!
27 July	Telephoned Clerk to chase letter of confirmation.
28 July	Received letter of confirmation.

The couple concluded their letter as follows:

> It has taken a lot of perseverance and determination during a period in excess of two years for us to get this far. We consider that the treatment we were given was disgraceful, especially the failure to notify us of our acceptance and would like to make an official complaint to the Ombudsman – but we are afraid to take any such action in fear of a reprisal (our chance of adoption might be taken away or at least delayed considerably).

This couple were very fortunate to receive a baby two years later, and this, in a sense, would have more than made up for the rather poor treatment they suffered from their Social Services Department. But far worse can happen.

My husband and I ... approached _____ Social Services in 1980. We were approved as adopters of a sibling group up to the age of about 9 in 1982 (eighteen months of tortuous procedures opening up old wounds which were far better left undisturbed, of if they must be so disturbed then why are those undergoing assessment left to wallow in distress without any counselling support?) However, we felt that in order for our goal to be reached we were willing to subject ourselves to this process. You can imagine ... how we felt in 1983 (exactly three years from the time we first approached _____ Social Services and after what we felt was a long time to wait for what we had been led to believe was a lengthy queue of needy children) on being told that ... 'approval doesn't necessarily mean that a child will be offered'. I ask, then, what does it mean? To say we felt shattered, betrayed, even raped, is to use words that are not really strong enough to describe our feelings. We withdrew, of course, and asked that our records be destroyed as by this time we had totally lost any trust in what had been written about us and did not want anyone else reading it.

Just as we were beginning to pick ourselves up we were approached by our local 'Be My Parent' agent informing us of the arrival of some new pages. We explained that we had withdrawn but she was very persuasive (how does one say 'no' to a child in need?) and we agreed to go and look. We found a 9-year-old boy from London, met his social worker who felt we had a lot to offer him but unfortunately the system demanded that as our papers had been destroyed (even though we produced our letter of acceptance) we would have to undergo the assessment procedure again and with no guarantee that this particular child would be assigned to us. This was in 1984 – more very difficult and painful decisions had to be made but

I for one was in no condition to go through that again without being interred in a mental hospital and I don't think our marriage would have stood the strain ...

It is now 1986 (six years from the time we first approached _____ Social Services) and I am only just now beginning to emerge and become able to talk about it ...

This woman has lost six years out of her life, and is only just beginning to recover from a most dreadfully painful experience. On the surface one could argue rationally that she and her husband should not have asked for their papers to be destroyed, but that would be to ignore the terrible distress that was caused at several stages of the adoption assessment process. And we are not dealing with someone who 'failed' to be selected, but with someone the authorities regarded as suitable to undertake a very special kind of adoption.

The assessment by a social worker of a couple's suitability to adopt is probably the most feared part of the whole adoption process. The couple are likely to worry about whether they will get on with the social worker or not, whether they will be able to create a favourable impression, what kind of personal questions they will be asked, and whether they will be able to cope when the social worker delves into the painful areas of their experience of infertility and how they feel about it. Above all, they have this fear that if they say or do the 'wrong' thing this one person alone has the power effectively to deny them their most cherished desire, to have a child of their own.

NAC receives many letters of complaint about the behaviour and attitudes of individual social workers towards the childless, and the 'brusqueness' of many social workers is commented on in research into this area.[15] Sometimes applicants feel that social workers are hostile to the childless. They may fear that the social worker will perceive them as people who 'expect other women to have babies for them', perceptions which are often fostered by sensational press coverage of topics such as surrogate mothering. They may be made to feel that they are wasting the social worker's time.

My goodness, I'd never met a social worker professionally before. Thank God I've never needed one. It would be like trusting your life to Lucrezia Borgia. We knew what to expect, we thought, because of that booklet on adoption. She just told us we were too old for that now and had we considered voluntary work with the aged!

A social worker came to see us. She was very sympathetic but she told us they had only placed three babies last year and had hundreds of people already on their list for any coming up. She said had we considered fostering, but we were so upset by what she'd told us we couldn't think of that at the time. Somehow, even though she was nice, she made us feel guilty about wanting to adopt a baby. We took up her time, we're trying to get in front of others in the queue. She didn't say this, but she implied it. When we said we'd never thought of fostering she lost all interest, it was as if we'd said no, when all we meant was we need time to think of it. Should we try again, or have we shot our bolt?

It took us two years to see the social worker about adoption. We kept writing every month or so. Eventually she came and we were ready, thanks to NAC. We'd read it all up. We'd thought about being willing to foster older children – we were. We'd thought of the problems. The first question she asked was whether we thought it was right to be asking. Had we not considered accepting our childlessness? Was adopting and fostering a solution really? I was mad. We'd thought this out carefully. Was she saying she thought we were unsuitable because we were childless? 'Oh no', she said, 'because you're in your late thirties and probably have got used to your situation without realising it.' I kept my head and told her we'd thought of that but felt we could do something useful by doing this and that we needed to change too. In the end, reluctantly, she filled in the form and took up our references. Now we have a lovely 10-year-old West Indian coming to us next week after several shorter stays. She didn't place him though. He came from a city, 40 miles away, who advertised. She never even told us we'd been accepted, or rejected, until the arrangements had been made with the other city.

This very limited survey of the adoption and fostering experience, from the point of view of the childless, has painted a very gloomy picture of both the present and likely future prospects for child adoption and fostering. Is there any way in which its administration could be improved, so that while the childless remain aware that their chances of success are necessarily small, they do feel that they are helped through the process by the social work profession and its bureaucracy, rather than hindered?

At the outset it has to be said that the sometimes appalling lengths of time that applicants have to wait for a decision as to whether they are approved or not surely requires investigation. It is difficult to know whether this is due to cumbersome bureaucracy, lack of resources, to adoption services being given a low priority, or to indifference on the part of the authority to the inconvenience and distress caused to those who apply. Surely it is possible to speed up the approval process.

We also wonder if some means of co-ordinating information between agencies can be developed, so that agencies whose lists are closed do not needlessly refer would-be applicants to other agencies whose lists are also closed. A great deal of time and wasted effort could be saved by all parties.

We also question whether the very low upper age limit for applications set by some agencies actually reflects the age distribution of the childbearing sector of the population. More and more professional women are starting their families after they enter their thirties, and continue to have children into their early forties. Imposing stringent age-limit rules does cut down the numbers of applicants to adoption agencies. But at the national level of broad policy formation, higher age limits would increase the pool of people available for fostering as well as adoption. Fewer people might also resort to practices such as surrogate mothering, which impose all kinds of legal and ethical problems. But this presupposes that adoption is looked at very broadly as part of childbearing and population planning strategy at a national level, which does not seem to be the case now.

Turning to the assessment of applicants' suitability to adopt, it is recognised that the formal requirements have to be carried out in the interests of all the parties, especially the interests of the child, but the present system of assessment is seen as very 'punitive' by many people. A very vulnerable group, the childless, are exposed to many of their most distressing feelings by a person they may not trust and whom they fear will not think well of them as a result. One possible solution would be the introduction of some kind of in-service training for adoption workers on the special needs of the childless. This would probably not require a great financial investment, and could possibly be covered in as little as a two-day workshop. An understanding of the needs of the childless is already incorporated into the practice of some social workers;[16] and there are many others who, through their sympathetic awareness of the suffering of the childless, do manage to help couples to understand their situation more fully, without the applicants officially becoming clients of the agency.

Greater sympathy and understanding might also enable social workers to persuade the childless to undertake a different form of parenting, which actually meets the needs of the agency and its clients, the children in need.

The social worker was really nice. It was a surprise. Ever so gently she told us about how few babies there were and suggested we might think about fostering an older child with a view to adoption. She knew that might be a shock to us and we might like time to think, so why didn't we fill in the application forms with her so we could at least start the process, and she'd come again in two weeks. She left us some booklets too. She said to phone her if we needed anything explaining. Well, we had a lot of questions when she came back and we talked it all over that time and then again a month later, when we agreed to go ahead. Eventually she introduced us to our first child placed with us. None of it's been easy, but we've been well served by this lady who understood us enough to help us be of use where we were needed.

Perhaps the most positive change would be a reassessment on the part of adoption agencies of their selection policy. It would seem that the assessment/selection model, whereby applicants are relegated to an inferior position at all stages of enquiries, might be better replaced by a preparation/education approach.[17] By this means, social workers work together with applicants, within a more equal relationship. Together they explore, over a period, the nature of what is required. There is much greater use made of group meetings with other applicants; and the intention is that over time applicants themselves are enabled to make their own decisions about whether adoption (or fostering) is appropriate for them. It is recognised that formal decisions still have to be made, but the process as a whole is likely to be much less harmful to the childless, as they will have more control and feel less helpless at most stages of the process.

However, what is needed most of all is a change of attitude towards the childless who seek to adopt. They are often made to feel that wanting a child of their own is an 'illegitimate' human desire; that people in their position should not be wasting time thinking about having babies, but should be making the best of the freedoms they have, by actively seeking alternatives. After all, they have been granted freedoms denied to those who have to bring up children. The woman of the partnership, in particular, is expected to appreciate the new role possibilities open to those women who choose not to have children, who refuse to take up the traditionally oppressed role of 'mother', perhaps motivated by the espousal of some form of feminist philosophy and politics. But to think in this way is to have a very limited understanding of what it means to be fully human, and of what constitutes woman's fully human activity. This is perhaps best expressed in the socialist feminist description of woman's activity given by Muriel Dimen:

> What we desire and need is not only 'to hunt in the morning, fish in the afternoon, rear cattle in the evening, criticise after dinner ... without ever becoming hunter, fisher ..., shepherd, or critic'. We also desire and need sometimes to cook and clean, sometimes to make babies and raise children, and often, spontaneously, to play with our

bodies, with ourselves, and with other women, men, and children, without even becoming 'only a housewife', somebody's mother, 'the head of the household', or perpetual children.

'Making babies' and 'raising children' are legitimate and genuine human aspirations and needs, and it is essentially good to want these experiences. If those who work with the childless could understand this, it would be of much comfort and support to them as they struggle to come to terms with the possibility that they may never have a child of their own.

This chapter, though concerned with adoption as a possible solution to childlessness, has attempted to show that it is becoming an increasingly unrealistic alternative for the majority of the childless. Though this will be regretted by many, it is not realistic, particularly for the older childless, to think that this situation will change for the better as a solution. The future does seem to lie with improved medical treatments, and for the many who, at present, are unable to benefit from these treatments, it is hoped that the following chapters will provide some solace, and help them in their long struggle towards adjustment and a new vision of the future.

11

Facing the need for acceptance

The present chapter looks at the experiences of childless people who have had to come to terms with their situation. It is when medical investigations have come to an end without a positive outcome, that the childless may be faced with the realisation that they can hope for nothing further from fertility treatments. They may then look for acceptable alternatives such as AID or adoption. If either or both of these fail, in the majority of cases it really is the end of the road as far as the possibility of having a child is concerned. Yet people differ to some extent as to when the acceptance process and the search for alternatives is actually considered to begin. For some childless women having a child means primarily bearing their own child by their husband or partner: 'The hospital also recommended that we start thinking about adoption as there is little chance of us having a baby of our own. We do not want to adopt a child and feel that we should not give up hope.'

Here we have a couple with negative feelings about adoption, and ideas about alternatives which conflict with those of their medical advisers. The hospital sees the fulfilment of its duty as advising the couple that pregnancy is not to be achieved, and that they should consider an alternative way to become parents. For the couple there is no alternative, although sometimes such a couple will later consider adoption. But for the present case we will assume that they do not. For them, the realisation of a need to accept their childless state would only begin when they could find no other medical help or were refused any further treatment. With the existence of the private sector, this couple could continue to seek medical help for several years if they could afford to pay. Thus 'the end of the road' is rather a subjective definition. The specialist defines it in terms of the results of a number of treatments which he or she believes to be reliable indicators of the ability of a couple to produce a baby. The childless may accept this definition, but refuse to believe that the medical assessment is correct. Adoption officers tend to use the medical definition. It is very common for them to be required to satisfy an adoption agency that an infertile couple 'has come to terms with their infertility', before accepting them as adoptive parents. This is a rather tricky phrase to understand, for if a couple have fully come to terms with their infertility or childlessness, it would seem unlikely that they would want to apply for adoption. In practice, the social worker uses certain observational criteria which suggest that the couple being investigated are reasonably emotionally balanced and have overcome the trauma of discovering their infertility.

Perhaps the nearest one can reach to a useful understanding as to when the process of 'coming to terms' begins, is to suggest that it starts when a couple or single person realises that they are unlikely to become parents in a way that is acceptable to them, and that as a consequence they will be forced to consider some other way to make their lives meaningful. Thus, some of the childless will see adoption or donor insemination as alternatives, which will require a great deal of thought and readjustment if they are to be considered or entered into. Others will make no distinction in their minds between the various available ways of becoming a parent, and for them the need to accept means the need to accept a childless future rather than the need to accept their personal infertility.

The present chapter is mainly concerned with the problems experienced by those who realise that their future is not going to be about the rearing of children, though it is hoped that it will also be of help to those who have children, but are still concerned about their infertility. For many of the involuntary childless, the mere thought of a future without children is too frightening to contemplate, and a flickering hope is maintained for many years before the possibility that there may be no children can be seriously entertained. The childless come to this realisation in different ways. As has been illustrated in earlier chapters, one common way for them to be forced to consider a childless future is at the termination of medical enquiries. It may be suggested to a couple, tactfully or bluntly, and it may sometimes be too much for them to cope with, so that they try to deny it or become exceedingly angry with the person who gave them the bad news. The overwhelming feeling is one of shock, from which the couple may take some time to recover. A failed adoption application may be another unpleasant experience which forces a couple to face the prospect of a very bleak future. In both these cases, it is an external source which challenges a couple's expectations about their future.

But many of the childless themselves also face the need for acceptance without it being suggested to them that they should. If medical and adoption enquiries have not had successful outcomes after a period of time, it may slowly become apparent to an individual or couple that the future might have to be faced without the prospect of children. It becomes necessary to consider this if there is to be any peace of mind, any rest after the long search. One NAC member wrote on her application form in the section headed 'Information required': 'Alternative lifestyles now that we shall not be having a family. Overcoming the depression.'

Another, less common, way to approach the need for acceptance of the childless state is for a couple to terminate all investigations of their own free will. This is not an easy decision to come to, particularly at present when so many 'miracle cures' appear to be available, from test-tube babies to yoghurt douches, cough mixtures and hormone pumps attached to the arm. But there *are* people who feel that stopping treatment at a particular point is the right decision for them. Naomi Pfeffer and Anne Woollett describe one woman's experience:

> *31 July 1980.* Period starts. I've run out of oestrogen tablets. The hospital no longer dispenses them so I have to go to my G.P. Since I moved I haven't found a new G.P. By the time I work all this out, it's too late to take Clomid this cycle.
>
> This summer is the third since we tried to conceive. We work on the house. I find out through my friend at the hospital that I do not have antibodies to Paul's sperm. It dawns on me that I have decided by default not to continue. The next test might be the one which gives me the answer. They might just find something that works for me. But then I remember what the tests were like, and I feel loath to go back to the hospital and try again.
>
> I feel the key question is changing slowly. I am asking less why am I infertile. Instead I am thinking about how to reconcile myself with my infertility and how I can move forward into a life in which children may not have a central role. I feel this is where I prefer to put my energies, and that continuing with the tests will interfere with this. So I do not go back to the clinic.[1]

The initial decision not to continue investigations is influenced here by the difficulties of obtaining treatment, which are caused by the cumbersome bureaucracy of the NHS. This is not an uncommon experience. The hospital system in general can act as a fairly effective deterrent:

> I went to the hospital for the last time yesterday. I don't see the point in continuing a fruitless trail. I was getting really depressed with the whole affair so I called a halt. I'm sure they don't really know what they're doing: they may know in theory but we ladies are much more complicated than that.

Among the childless who are going through medical tests, the frustration and disappointment leading to a decision to discontinue investigations are easily understood. But a decision to discontinue, or reject, donor insemination appears more threatening, both to those who support it, and those who reject it. A member of NAC wrote to the newsletter:

> As the day of reckoning drew near, we both became more and more uneasy and finally came to the conclusion that AID was not the answer for us.
>
> I can't explain the wonderful feeling of tranquillity that came over me as I ceremoniously ripped up my temperature charts and other bits and pieces. Of course we will never be able to blot out the last two years, but the change that has come over us as a couple is quite noticeable, I think. We are almost light-hearted again and time will, I expect, heal most of the pain.

This letter appeared side by side with letters describing successful donor insemination experiences; and it is interesting that the woman who had decided against donor insemination felt that her brave decision had to be justified in the light of the evidence which seemed to downgrade her experience. The next issue of *NACK* contained a further letter from her giving detailed reasons for her and her husband's decision not to proceed with donor insemination. It is possible that other members who knew her had voiced their disagreement. It is also possible that the whole area of artificial insemination by donor is so fraught with unresolved guilt feelings imposed by the need for secrecy, that it brings to the fore feelings of deep unease (in the same way as can happen with abortion). Diane herself remembers a NAC meeting several years ago where she talked about coming to terms with childlessness, and mentioned, almost in passing, that she considered donor insemination wrong for herself, and gave reasons for this. Several people failed to listen to a word after that. In the ensuing question period she was attacked for her decision. Yet she had not said donor insemination was wrong, only that it would have been wrong for her. There was a need for these people to justify their involvement with the donor insemination process, but it was not necessary. They were not being attacked. It is to be hoped that the legal and ethical problems posed by donor insemination can be ultimately resolved, so that those who decide both for it and against it can receive social support for their decision, particularly from other childless people.

There is a third way in which the childless may be brought face to face with the need to consider a future without children. That is when the age of the woman makes is seem unlikely that she will become pregnant. In the past, adoption would have been an alternative possibility in such a case, even for a single woman under certain circumstances. It is difficult at the present time to ascertain at what age a woman comes into the third category. Some doctors set age limits for carrying out complex surgical techniques such as *in-vitro* fertilisation. The operation does not have a successful record with women over 40, and 36 is the preferred maximum age for the techniques by some specialists. Yet cases are recorded of women giving birth in their late forties, and thus it is difficult to decide when a woman should consider herself beyond the fertile years if she is in good health and still having monthly periods. A few much younger women would belong in this category if they have had an early menopause or a hysterectomy, and are not eligible to apply for adoption, because, for example, an adoption agency has set a fairly low upper age limit for eligibility, say the age of 33. Thus the age at which it seems unreasonable for a woman to hope for pregnancy or adoption will be determined by a variety of factors, and women themselves may give widely differing ages when asked this question. The most that can be said is that is would be difficult to find anyone who thought that a woman had a chance of conceiving or adopting at the age of 50 or above.

If one turns to the reconciliation process itself, and asks whether any of the factors discussed above have any impact on the ability of a couple or single person to adapt successfully to life without the prospect of children, it is difficult to make generalisations. Deciding for oneself rather than being told might be an initial help, but people do get over the initial distress of being told in an unsympathetic way. Age, too, is not crucial. The NAC files show people under twenty-five who have made the decision to accept life without children. There are also people in their late forties and older who write in to enquire about the possibilities of having a child. There are also women without a partner who hope for a baby, possibly by donor insemination. The source of the need to come to terms, a woman's age, and marital status, are less important than a number of other factors which will be discussed in the next section. And, as has been said, a certain number of people who have adopted, or are secondarily infertile, will also have a need for acceptance of their infertility.

Three case studies

In order to decide if there are any important factors which influence the way a childless person is able to accept his or her condition, and achieve a reasonably satisfactory life, let us look at the responses of three women in very different circumstances, who all face a childless future. Let us call them Angela, Celia and Mrs Wood. They have three things in common – they are over forty, they have all been married for some time, and none of them knows the cause of their infertility, though they have all undergone medical investigations in the past. Beyond this, they respond to their situation in very different ways.

Angela is 42, and her husband 46. They have lived for some years on an estate where the majority of couples have children. After medical investigations lasting five years, Angela was told by the specialist that there was nothing he could find wrong with her, and she should accept her infertility as God's will. Possibly because of her very insecure childhood, leading to much unhappiness later on, she and her husband were turned down for adoption or fostering. They feel very isolated socially and at work, where, Angela writes, 'I feel a failure never having conceived, and one feels inferior when all these women talk about their children.' If she mentions her childlessness they all pity her, or say how lucky she is to be free. She follows TV and radio soap operas to have a family that she can feel part of, and once tried to be an Aunty at a children's home, but sensed that she was not wanted.

Angela knows that she must come to terms with her situation, but finds this hard:

> I accept it is God's will that I cannot change circumstances, but I should like to know how to get on top and cope with them better, as sometimes I get quite despairing and depressed and when, basically, our 15 years of married life have been sort of the same and without the changes of growing families, the future must be worked at.

The greatest problem for Angela and her husband seems to be social isolation:

> We find we seem to be outside everyone's circle. We have no close family and find all our acquaintances are fully involved with their family life, by now most with teenagers and newly-wed in-laws and the new grandchildren. We help with Save-the-Children Fund and I have also with other charities. My husband works full-time, I part-time. We belong to quite a lot of groups and have a variety of interests, but we find wherever we go and whoever we talk to their families *quite naturally* fill their lives, come uppermost in their thoughts and experiences. I know of only two (older) couples in this vicinity without children. One says she loves her job too much to give up and have children, and the other one seems completely fulfilled making a full-time job of cooking and housework.

This couple illustrate very clearly the problems of peripherality described in chapter eight. Although they have relationships with many different people in different situations, they generally feel excluded from the social interaction through their lack of a family. They feel peripheral – on the outside, looking in.

Celia is very different from Angela. She has been an art teacher for many years, and has exhibited her own work. Recently she took over her parents' business. Her husband is a lecturer. They had both adjusted to a life without children many years before NAC came into being, yet chose to join the Association shortly after its founding:

> We have followed the Association's progress with great interest in the press and on radio. You have done something very positive in bringing this issue out into the open for general discussion. When we were contending with our fertility about eighteen years ago, the climate was very different. Though we had one of the great experts in the field, in this area, to take regular clinics – I always had to go to the Family Planning Clinic and wait *hours* with women all lining up for contraceptives! I often wondered then – as we both did – whether it might have been best to leave the problem alone. I found the whole process distressing – and I don't think it need have been. However, life streams take one on, and we learn to accept all things as time reveals the pattern.

For Celia, now 47, life is meaningful within the terms of her personal philosophy:

> The great advantage of becoming older is that one – hopefully – becomes more philosophical – more 'supple' in one's thoughts. It is not easy to achieve this, though, as well I know. But as years go by one is presented with wider vistas, full of possibilities.

Accompanying one of her letters to the Association is a photo of Celia, in her shop, holding a friend's baby. It is one of those pictures that compels one to look at it again, and again. It is not because of the baby. It is Celia. The warmth of her smile, her vitality, make one think 'I would like to know this woman'. One could say that she has a beautiful aura.

There is no picture of *Mrs Wood*. She is *Mrs* Wood because she does not reveal her first name. She and her husband are now 50 and they live in a traditionally conservative part of Britain. They have been married for well over twenty years. She has a clerical job, and he works for one of the public services. Since the age of 46, Mrs Wood has been writing to NAC at regular intervals, asking for information about different methods of obtaining a child. Her letters are always polite, to the point, asking for help, but revealing nothing about herself that would enable one to form some kind of mental image of her. There are no small details that would enable the reader to decide what sort of life she led, whether she had any friends or relatives, nothing to show how her husband felt about having no children.

At 46 she writes in connection with her attempts to be accepted for *in-vitro* fertilisation:

> As you may remember I told you in my last letter that I had written to Mr ——'s secretary, but they do not accept anybody over the age of 36 years, unfortunately I am quite a long way over the age limit, being 46 years.
>
> I would have thought they would have given older people the option to decide for themselves, as time is against them.

She finds another specialist, and writes: 'I wrote to Mr ——, but he regretfully does not operate on anyone over the age of 45. I don't suppose you have any more addresses I might try.' Another name was given to her:

> I did contact Dr ——, but he regretfully said I would have to come to terms with my not being able to have any children.
>
> I do not think anyone is willing to take the risk with older people. If you should at any time know of anyone who would consider me for a test-tube baby, please let me know. I do not have time to wait unfortunately.
>
> P.S. I do not mind adopting a child up to about 5 years.

She then joins NAC, and under the heading 'Information required', puts:

> Adoption.
> (1) Abroad or in this country. It may be time consuming and expensive, but we should like the opportunity, please, of trying to adopt from another country.
>
> We don't want any literature forwarded to us. Please do not think we are awkward, but it is only how we can get into contact in this country or abroad we are interested in.

Secrecy is vital. They would not like their affairs known locally. But her adoption enquiries are not successful. She writes a few months later: 'There must be a child somewhere I could adopt and give a good home to.' A few months after this she writes in again for new information:

> I am 47 years of age, but I am still having periods and am quite healthy and young in outlook. So could you please give me the address of someone responsible who would consider my husband and I for AIH. Please help us as we have no time to waste. I will gladly pay.

A year later she is still concerned to adopt: 'Please help me, as I am getting older, and my chances are slipping away. I just do not have the time to waste.' Eighteen months on she writes of the depths of her desire for a child:

> My husband and I are both 49 years of age and of course I would have liked to have had a child of my own but was not able to, and the older you get the longing gets more and more. I had thought some marvellous discovery could be made whereby people of my age could still have a child – but it seems impossible. But that is my dearest wish.

A month later she asks for more information about adoption: 'My husband and I will be 50 years old this year and I know it is going to be very difficult for us to adopt so we would like all the help that you are able to give.'

On my forty-third birthday, writing this chapter of our book, I put down my pen, and wept for Mrs Wood. I wept for a woman whose face was unknown to me, a woman nursing a secret sorrow, who did not want to be known. And I picked a Peace rose from the garden, to console us both.

What makes the response of these three women to a similar situation so different? With the limited information available it is difficult to make any judgments with certainty. But there are some possible pointers enabling one to make some tentative comments. Angela, it would appear, lives in a rather difficult environment for a sensitive childless person. She and her husband are surrounded by people whose social lives are dominated by family concerns. One would also guess that Angela lacks confidence in herself, probably because of past experiences. Yet she is aware of her own problems, and able to describe them clearly. Someone like Angela might benefit from being in touch with NAC Contacts, who would listen to her patiently, and encourage her when she feels most depressed. She and her husband might make some more congenial friendships if there are activities for NAC members in their area. Angela would perhaps be able to cope better with conversations about children if she had more confidence in herself; if there were an appropriate local counselling service, she might benefit from some sort of professional help. It is likely that she will always find life somewhat hard, but she has the courage to get out and try to make a go of things, and one would want to wish for a less troubled life for her and her husband.

When we turn to Celia, it becomes evident that we are dealing with a very talented and articulate woman. Many of the feelings that she would have expressed towards children, if she and her husband had been able to have them, have gone into her teaching, painting, social life and activities in her business. She and her husband have a clear understanding of what their problem is, and are able to reason through it philosophically. Because she feels at home with her own personality, she is able to show generosity towards others. There are not too many Celias around.

What can one say about Mrs Wood? It is difficult, as she says so little about herself. We know nothing of what her husband feels about having or not having children. One could perhaps guess that the part of the country in which Mrs Wood lives makes it very difficult for her to admit that she is infertile, and that her neighbourhood does not encourage women to have any ambitions beyond having a family. Her job, too, is not at all creative, and would be unlikely to provide her with any emotional outlet. Like Angela, one might feel that Mrs Wood lacks self-confidence. But what is the source of that deep longing for a child, that will not leave her? It is hard to say. Perhaps being a mother is the one thing in life she would have been happy with, and good at. Nothing in her experience so far has come anywhere near it. Has she accepted that she is very unlikely ever to have a child? It is difficult to say. Common sense suggests that she may have, but what is the nature of that acceptance? We do not know. She lives hoping against all hope.

How is reconciliation achieved?

Not a great deal is known about the way in which a childless person comes to terms with his or her childless state, and is enabled to work towards an alternative view of life, or a lifestyle that offers some of the rewards that are comparable to those experienced in the bearing or bringing up of children. Many of the medical texts on infertility contain sections on coming to terms, or alternative lifestyles, but such a section is generally brief in comparison with the rest of the book. There are some good accounts of the emotional component of fertility investigations, but we do not know of any detailed studies that attempt to investigate the way in which reconciliation comes about in practice.[2] Thus there is a need for research into this process, including investigations of the factors that make it easier or less easy for a person to make the necessary adjustment; and also for some indications of the types of experience likely to be encountered on the way, and the more effective ways of dealing with such experiences.

The present work can, therefore, only be based on a survey of the recorded accounts of those NAC members who have felt that they should write about their experiences subsequent to discovering their infertility, plus insights gained from our own personal experiences. Many NAC members discontinue their links with the Association once they have reached some kind of reconciliation. This would appear to be quite natural, and must be regarded as a step forward in the adjustment process. Telephone counselling and visits of NAC Contacts would be an alternative source of information about the nature of the process, but much of this work is of necessity confidential. The following account attempts to set the scene for more detailed investigations, which we hope will be undertaken by interested researchers in the future.

It must be said that not every person without children in adult life goes through this process. It is doubtful whether people whose lives are so ordered that they would not naturally have children (e.g. religious orders, single people) can all be considered to need to go through the reconciliation process. An essential requirement for beginning the process has to be a recognition that a personal need exists to make the necessary adjustment. This recognition may not be perceived as such at the time by the individuals concerned. It may only be apparent in retrospect, many years later, when people look back over their past experiences and try to make sense of them. But with advances in medical techniques, and the gradual disappearance of adoption as a way to have children of one's own, it is likely that the involuntary childless will become more aware of the need to rethink their life objectives.

Not only must the childless feel the need to come to terms with infertility but they must also be prepared to do something about that need. A little faith in the ability of the individual to accept change will help, but is not essential. Just being aware is a good start:

> I feel at the moment that I am at the end of the road, so to speak, entering 'the final phase of acceptance' and yet because I have never found out the reason for my infertility, I wonder whether I ever will be able to totally accept it. I must sound rather confused – but I must admit, I do feel very confused right now. If only we could be told a reason, something positive then I'm sure the business of getting down to accepting the situation would be much easier.

Admission of the existence of a problem seems, in some miraculous way often to enable the brain to begin its work of problem solving. A new perception may be triggered off, some time later, by an external event or experience There is an example of this on page 66, where a woman describes her distress on hearing of the birth of Prince William: 'I suddenly found myself unable to hold in my feelings any longer and sobbed uncontrollably for half an hour. I felt the heartbreak of years flooding out and I know it was healing.'

Another woman wrote in to NAC to discontinue her membership:

> I certainly was in a bad way a year or less ago. I couldn't bear to watch children, to visit anyone who had children, even to hear anyone talk about their children; the whole world seemed sometimes to conspire to make me remember that I was being deprived of the one thing I wanted more than anything else... it wasn't helped by the fact that my specialist couldn't think of any reason why I wasn't ovulating, or of any treatment except Clomid, which had no effect at all.
>
> The change came quite suddenly, in a moment of what I can only describe as God-given insight. 'Ah, my trouble isn't that I can't get pregnant – my trouble is that I am *upset* at not getting pregnant. And *that* is something I can do something about.'

Here the trigger event is not known, but it would seem that the hopelessness of the medical investigations had slowly dawned on the writer over a period of time, and her solution came to her almost as a miracle at the moment when her mind had sufficient understanding for the work of healing to begin.

On other occasions people may have perceptions that the work of reconciliation has already begun without their realising it. Each issue of *NACK* contains a short article on pets by Brenda Holliday, which is popular with many members. One woman, married to a tetraplegic, described how she had been helped by her pets.

> Recently I was feeling particularly depressed about our childless state and was on the verge of tears, when I heard Joey saying 'Who's a naughty boy,' 'Joey a pretty boy,' 'Put the kettle on.' In came the dogs, Pip with his head on my lap offering sympathy, and Rover with his lead in his mouth reminding me they had not had their walkies yet. I suddenly realised I had a smile on my face and was feeling a whole lot better, refreshed as if I had just sat and talked to some sympathetic friend.
>
> I leapt from my chair, tried to have a chat with Joey, amidst his own line of chatter. Thought about getting Toby a nice female cockatiel with whom perhaps he can perform his duties successfully. The dogs and I went up on the moors with our picnic lunches, and had a joyous afternoon on our own away from normality, so to speak.
>
> I can honestly say, I felt so much better for the pets, and had not realised up to then, how amazingly they seemed to realise how much their owner needed sympathy and understanding in a time of despair and they were there readily offering their all to help. Malcolm and I would not part with our pets for all the 'tea in China' and enjoy every moment we have with them.

The importance of the above experience does not lie in the events, but in the meaning interpreted from them by the individual concerned. It is the interpretation of what has happened that is crucial. This is important to understand if one is to become involved in counselling the childless, or offering professional advice. There can be no generally valid rules about those things it is necessary for the childless to do, or ways in which they should think or feel. Time, the great healer, performs part of the process.

Sympathy, interest and the ability of the counsellor to listen and encourage are another part. Sometimes it will be appropriate to suggest ideas or activities. But the most important and influential suggestions are likely to be those that the childless person initially believes to have come from himself or herself. What is suggested has to be in tune with the individual's disposition, talents and circumstances. Interestingly, many of the trigger events appear to have taken place within the framework of everyday life and routines. The first recognition of the possibility of a solution perhaps needs some form of security in which to develop. It is later on that the bigger changes may be relevant, and can then be suggested.

Once there is an awareness, supported by some kind of personal insight that it may be possible to think or live in a different way, the healing process can start. It is, in many cases, a lengthy process, and not always a straightforward progression. There may be several false starts, or steps backward. It is both an internal and external process, each aspect reinforcing the other. Several bad experiences may lead to a loss of some of the confidence newly gained, but in general something essentially good is retained from earlier insights, and it is possible for people to recover with help and encouragement.

The adjustment required is often very demanding, in terms of the intellectual and emotional engagement needed. Sometimes the body has also to play a part in the process. This is true with, for example, women who have had a miscarriage, a hysterectomy or early menopause. The experience of discovering one is infertile may also exact a toll on one's physical health. Depression can be very debilitating, as can loss of sexual libido, loss of confidence in oneself as an acceptable person, and anger and bitterness. Any or all of these may be present in the initial stages of coming to terms with childlessness. It must be borne in mind, then, that the healing process may require very extensive investment, and the practitioner who is likely to be of most help in this respect is one who is able to deal with the childless person as a human being with complex and inter-related needs. These needs will be looked at in some detail in the following chapter.

12

Assisting the healing process

In this chapter we shall look at some possible solutions to problems encountered by the childless, as they attempt to adjust to the prospect of a life without children. Three important areas will be considered:

(i)   dealing with medical aspects
(ii)   coping with feelings
(iii) making decisions

Though the physical, emotional and social aspects will be covered separately, for ease of understanding, it should be borne in mind that all three may be related to each other in complex ways, and each will influence the others in the healing process.

Medical aspects

One fairly common problem, for those who decide that they should try to come to terms with their childless state, is how and when to terminate medical investigations. Although the childless often seem to be disappointed with the standard of medical care given, the 'helpful specialist' can also present them with problems. It is not easy to call a halt to treatment if the doctor or specialist is committed to a policy of 'success at almost any cost'. Kindness and enthusiasm may be more difficult to counter than brusqueness or indifference, because the latter do enable the childless to shift the burden of the decision onto other people. It sometimes seems easier to claim that one stopped treatment because of the rudeness or incompetence of Dr X, than to admit to having doubts about the treatment offered by pleasant, competent Dr Y.

There is also another reason why some people find it difficult to discontinue treatment. In the quotation on page 118 from the book by Naomi Pfeffer and Anne Woollett, the problem is seen clearly. There was the feeling that by making a definite decision to discontinue treatment, one might miss something vital: 'The next test might be the one which gives me the answer. They just might find something that works for me.'[1] A breathing space, suggested either by the specialist or the patient, might be an acceptable solution for both parties. The woman in chapter one who gave up taking Bromocriptine, and then went back on to it two years later at a lower dose, to achieve a successful pregnancy, solved the problem one way. The woman in Naomi Pfeffer and Anne Woollett's book solved it by stopping treatment altogether, making a determined effort to adjust to a new view of herself and to move into a life where children would not have a central role. It does need to be stressed, however, that it is not easy to know whether the correct decision has been made, and there will probably be a certain amount of agonising before coming to terms with that decision, whether it is to continue or discontinue treatment.

There are several circumstances where the decision to stop treatment may be necessitated by an existing medical condition, an inability to carry a pregnancy to full term, or a risk to the health of the baby. There are also medical conditions where the health of the mother would be seriously at risk, and the specialist may feel that pregnancy should be discouraged. Early hysterectomy and early menopause are other medical conditions which effectively take the decision to continue treatment out of the hands of the patient. People in these categories may have extra problems to cope with, and need great courage and much support if they are to pull through.[2] Lynne Pemberton described her reaction on hearing that she had cancer: 'I was completely numb. Before the phone went down I was in tears and sure I was going to die. The first thing I thought of was, I can't have children. The fact that it was cancer hit me about 30 seconds later.'[3]

Sometimes those who suffer from a medical condition affecting their ability to become pregnant, receive well-meaning but misguided 'help'. It can be very damaging to be forced to face one's infertility, and then have one's hopes falsely raised:

I am writing in the hope that you can help me. In June of 1980 after four years of infertility investigations, I was diagnosed as having a premature menopause. In December 1981 this was confirmed by an independent gynaecologist.

I am now 32 years of age and have adjusted to the prospect of a life without children and hormone replacement therapy for the rest of my life. (Does anyone *ever* adjust?) Then Bang! All my family and friends are telling me about a TV programme that went out on the 'air' about a month ago. The programme referred to a new infertility treatment which involved hormone doses measured and issued by a 'pack' strapped to the arm. The treatment is new but seems to have a high success rate for women who fail to ovulate or who have never ovulated.

One of the success cases was a woman who had been diagnosed as menopausal at 23. As I did not see the programme the above details are sketchy, but I feel I must follow this up. Can you help me in any way?

This letter was referred to the NAC medical advisers. Their comments on the treatment were that its success was much over-rated. It could only help a small percentage of women, and was still fairly experimental. Anyway it cannot help in the menopause.

A rather different medical problem, often connected with unsuccessful infertility investigations, is that of depression. There are no statistics as to how common it is amongst those experiencing infertility, but it is frequently mentioned by those coming to the end of medical treatment, and those attempting to adjust to a life without children. In general, depression does seem to be a problem experienced more by women, for a variety of reasons, and in different situations. It may be related to the inability of many women to express their real feelings, as suggested by Veronica Horwell:

> For it was isolation that caused it. Not loneliness – some depressed women are never let, or let to be, *alone* – but a remoteness. We are connected to humanity through our faults and feelings, and when we have no-one to tell about these, or trust no-one enough to share with them the truth, or even suppress them from ourselves, then the communications systems are down.

> All the women I know who have passed over into depression had kept their real selves at a distance. They projected a perfect and immobile creation – often a huge caricature – Mrs Composure, Miss Compassionate, Mrs Hostess and Mother of Three – while their imperfect and changing originals were slumped inside without an outside line to anyone.

For Veronica Howell, depression was a big black dog padding behind her. She describes her final encounter with it:

> I began to understand that he would always be there unless I turned and faced him, actively changed my life. I would have to accept the emotions I ignored, hate and love, get involved where I had been aloof, make friends, not acquaintances. I should have to leave my secure boring job and my safe house, jump out of the riskless but gloomy trench I had dug for myself, yell at people, ladder my tights, miss the last tram and the last plane, take a chance on chaos.[4]

Sometimes a childless person is so depressed that medical treatment is required, in order that distressing physical and mental symptoms may be brought under control, to enable the necessary reflection upon unresolved problems to begin. There is sometimes a fear of taking psychotropic or mood-altering drugs prescribed by a doctor. Some fear they will become addicted to the drugs, others feel they are being 'fobbed off' by the doctor – he or she is seen to be taking the easy way out by writing a prescription. Some of the childless get themselves into a state where they realise that they are depressed or anxious because of their infertility, but their mind tells them that they cannot take any of the pills prescribed for them, just in case the pills affect their chance of becoming pregnant.

It is true that the minor tranquillisers, in particular, are often prescribed as a drug of first resort, in some cases irresponsibly, and long-term use may lead to rare cases of addiction. It is also true that drugs alone will not banish any serious unresolved problems. But those who fear that the use of drugs for mental relief will adversely affect their fertility need to consider that stress, anxiety, fear and depression may also make it more difficult for a woman to conceive. It is all a question of balance. Responsibly prescribed, and accompanied by sympathetic counselling, minor tranquillisers and anti-depressant drugs, taken in accordance with the doctor's instructions, can make a considerable difference to a person's state of mind, giving one confidence to try and grapple with the problems causing the symptoms. The two types of drug mentioned above have very different functions, even though they are sometimes prescribed at the same time. If one is not sure which type of drug has been prescribed, it is best to ask the doctor rather than listen to old wives' (or husbands') tales. There are, however, one or two reasonably accurate books on drugs written for the general public, which can be very helpful, provided one does not immediately begin to experience every side-effect listed for each drug used![5] A final warning does need to be given for those who choose to reject drugs prescribed for them, because they feel that to take them is an admission of failure: 'Certainly in Western Society the puritan ethic of "being firm and standing on one's own two feet" may produce awful feelings of guilt and unworthiness in which suicide appears to be the only way out.'[6]

Some find relief in alternative medicine. If the products or methods used are known to be harmless, it does not matter whether they are accepted or discredited by the orthodox medical profession. Different methods of healing and spiritual disciplines 'work' for many people, and that is the most important thing. But it should also be remembered that if one is bitten by a poisonous snake, the prayers of one's friends will not save one from death. A serum antidote might.

Coping with feelings

Coping with one's feelings and making decisions are closely related in the healing process. Each reinforces the other, internally within the mind of the individual, and externally in relationships with the outside world. But it is important to understand one's own feelings before any decisions are made about changes likely to have a major impact on one's life.

The childless who are in the process of discovering that they may need to adjust to a life largely without children need to undertake some kind of assessment of their present feelings. Those who have supportive partners may be able to undertake this together. They should first ask what having a baby or child has meant to them. There are all kinds of answers that can be given to this question, some of them seemingly rather strange, but none of them wrong in themselves. Cuddling a small and beautiful creature, showing one's love for one's partner, making one's parents happy, being able to lift up one's head with one's friends, are just a few of the possible answers. The second question to be asked is how one generally feels in relation to the society of which one is a member. Some may want to feel acceptable or useful, others may want to take some kind of leadership role, others to sit on the side and watch. It is possible that one's relationship to society is quite complex and one may find that several different answers all seem correct. The third question to ask is – which aspects of one's present life still seem satisfactory, despite one's disappointment at not having a child? There may be many people and things that are still capable of giving pleasure and interest, or evoking feelings of love and understanding; one's partner, parents, relatives, friends, or work, hobbies, home, environment, travel, study, holidays, pets.... If, for any reason, it is difficult to give a positive answer to this question, whether the problem is due to social or economic conditions, or personal despair, it would be wise to seek outside help. But, hopefully, most people will be able to answer this question positively.

Taking time to consider the questions posed in the last paragraph should enable an individual or couple to have at least a very general idea of how they feel about life, and this represents a step forward in the process of adjustment. It is likely, however, that over the years of fertility investigations and hopes for a child, a residue of very negative feeling has built up, that acts as a hindrance to further adjustment. Many feelings of disappointment, anger, distrust and bitterness may need to be dissipated before one can view the world positively again.

Sometimes an incident or remark may evoke such strong feeling that all one's emotions burst out. Though it may be distressing at the time, it can provide a release for all those trapped, negative feelings that are slowly eating one up. Tears shed for some deep sorrow can be very healing, and in many ways it is a pity that our society discourages any too public display of emotion. People can needlessly inhibit themselves for years, as a result of a belief that it is wrong to give vent to strong feelings.

Where deep feelings are inadequately understood, dreams may sometimes provide some kind of release. One childless woman was able to recall a dream that helped her to face her condition, and understand her response to it:

> The figure suddenly disappeared into the Hall, which was very ornate indeed, as though on loan from Disney World, and appeared on a balcony looking shy and fragile. I turned to a local and asked if he knew what UMA meant. 'Oh, yes,' he said, 'its Czech for unborn child.' 'Oh', I said, rather startled and looking round again saw UMA coming out on the pavement dancing, whirling and embracing people. UMA was soon in front of me face to face, and what a face, but a familiar one in its sweet ugliness.

Diane, too, on one occasion, came to understand more about herself through a dream. She often dreamt of entering an unknown house, furnishing it, extending it and moving in. In one dream she found her country cottage and set about altering it as usual. She looked round the side, and saw that there was a problem. The cottage backed onto a sandy beach, so it was not possible to extend it. But when she looked round the back she saw that it was built into a rock. Though the house was limited by its surroundings, it was firm and secure against storms and the sea. Like the man who built his house on a rock 'And the rains descended and the floods came, and the winds blew and beat upon that house; and it fell not: for it was founded upon a rock.'[7]

It is sometimes helpful, in coming to terms with one's feelings, to hear the stories of others who have been through similar situations. Realising that someone else has felt the same way in comparable experiences can bring release. There is often guilt about negative thoughts that have been allowed to surface, and to suddenly see that what one has felt is fairly common under the circumstances enables one to place the negative feelings in their appropriate context. The damaging effect of these feelings may thereby be lessened.

The release of repressed emotions, the healing work of dreams, the realisation that one has experienced a known problem, all allow the individual to understand herself or himself better. The way in which these three operate may appear rather strange at times, as if they are not completely under one's control. But there are other negative emotions that may be very deeply buried, and are the result of an accumulation of many negative experiences. They may not be so accessible to any of the above methods of release, and may have to be worked on over a considerable period of time before they can be controlled and transformed into their positive correlatives.

Jealousy is a rather common emotion that is potentially destructive of relationships with others and their children. Sometimes the childless are aware that they are jealous of, perhaps, a relative's baby. If one understands more about the way the modern family tends to function, it may be easier to overcome jealousy of another who has a child. The present conception of the family in most of Western society is increasingly that of the nuclear family of two parents and (usually) two dependant children. With increasing isolation from other generations and branches of the family, the responsibility for the upbringing of the children falls more and more into the hands of the parents. Grandparents now have relatively little influence on the way their grandchildren are brought up. They interfere with daughter or daughter-in-law's child-rearing practices at their peril. The mother, in particular, assumes a greater responsibility for all aspects of the child's welfare, including the physical. As children, we both remember it was common for young girls in the street to offer to take a neighbour's baby for a walk in the pram. (Diane still remembers the commotion when they couldn't decide whether her younger brother had been left in Margaret Chicken's or Margaret's chickens!) As far as one can tell, this practice is less frequent now – the responsible mother may be frightened that the neighbour's daughter will let the baby be kidnapped, or drop it in the pond. Thus there is an increasing tendency towards a very possessive type of relationship towards the child, on the part of the parent. This possessiveness is socially accepted, and implicitly defines the boundaries of any relationship that other adults are allowed to have with the child. It makes it very difficult for the childless to have an appropriate relationship with someone else's child. The experience of the two teachers in chapter nine is a good illustration of the type of difficulty that can arise if the childless try to have a close relationship with a child, without the backing of those adults considered most responsible for the child.

The childless may need to realise that they are not going to be able to have the possessive type of relationship with children that is typical of many parents. They have to learn to disperse their love and affection over many people. This is not an easy thing to do. Indeed, some parents fail to realise that there are limits to the possessive relationship, even when their children are grown up. Thus it is likely to be extra difficult for those who have never had their own family, who have not experienced an intimate, protective love for someone small and defenceless, and totally under their control.

How can one learn that selfless love that responds to the needs of the other, rather than the needs of the giver? It is doubtful whether most ordinary mortals ever do learn it. The way towards it is long and hard, and involves total surrender of the self. It is not, therefore, very helpful to the childless to think that they can attain such heights. What they need to understand is how they, individually, can best cope with the problems posed by the need to disperse their affections. One way is to work through formal or informal situations where it is possible to extend one's affection to many, and yet difficult to have too intimate a relationship with one individual. Many jobs involving a pastoral relationship with children or adults would come into this category, as would work in many voluntary organisations. The person who has an understanding of his or her emotional needs, and who also implicitly recognises where the boundaries of a relationship should lie, may still be able to have a successful relationship with a child. There is great joy in being an aunt or uncle, or a godparent, provided one does not allow one's love and affection to lead to an attachment that demands unrealistic returns from the child. Others use the love that would have been given to a child for different creative purposes. A beautiful garden is a work of love; so is any craft or skill that attempts to transform ordinary, unremarkable materials into a work of art, which is a gift. Some people are able to use all three ways of dispersing their affections, and keep a balance between them that enables them to find a positive meaning to their lives. Celia, who was described in chapter ten, is an illustration of someone who has found a variety of ways to express some of the love that would have gone to her own children, if she had been able to have them.

When one understands that one is jealous of the opportunity given to others to possess, and that one would also like to possess, it becomes easier to accept that there have to be other ways to give and receive love; and it has been suggested that there are alternative ways to form relationships that many may find rewarding. Once this is understood, there may be yet another feeling on the part of the childless that needs to be looked at. But it is a feeling that is not in itself at all bad or unrealistic. The childless may look at the relationships that certain parents have with their children, and think, 'Given the chance, I could make a better job of bringing up those children than their parents have done.' It is true that some parents seem well qualified to mess up the lives of their children, and the newspapers love to report the sordid details of child cruelty cases. It is very hard for the childless to sit and watch an adult who takes delight in humiliating a child, or who is completely insensitive to a child's emotional needs. Yet there is not a lot that the observer can do, unless the cruelty is of such magnitude that it warrants legal intervention. Here the legitimation of possession is very much evident – one can do to one's children all kinds of things that would not be at all acceptable if one was responsible for other people's children. Thus it is hard for the childless to feel that their love and understanding have no place. But they do need to learn that it is not very helpful to them to compare their own parenting skills with other peoples'. Unless one has actually brought up a child one can never really know whether one would have been successful or not. One may have all the necessary qualities, but one will not be judged on preliminary qualifications, but on performance and results, and the judgments are likely to be subjective. No two parents have the same views as to what constitutes good childcare, and very often what works with one child may not be helpful to another. The childless need to learn to be more tentative in their views of their potential abilities as parents. It may be difficult to learn tolerance in provocative situations, but it has to be learnt if one is to continue good relationships with friends and relatives who have had children.

In the same way that a childless person needs to cope with his or her feelings towards other people, so do other people need to learn to cope with the sensitivities of the childless – in theory. In practice both friends and relatives can easily make hurtful remarks, whether intentional or not. The onus again seems to lie with the childless to make the adjustment. It is hard to learn not to be harmed by every ignorant or foolish statement. But it may be helpful to assume that most remarks are not meant to hurt. In many cases the opposite is indeed intended. Groups of women at work, for example, may talk a lot about their families. But this is often some kind of social code, the purpose of which is to extend and maintain goodwill, and by asking after someone's children one is doing just this. It may be noticed that the women find someone else to ask about if a woman has no children. It may be a husband, an aunt or a friend, even a pet. In a supportive group it may take some time to discover who has or does not have children.

It would seem that a great deal is demanded of the childless if they are to cope with the negative feelings and responses that make it difficult for them to overcome their sadness and isolation. Understanding oneself, and changing the way that one looks at the world, are part of a very long-term process of adjustment, and require both courage and flexibility. The adjustment may influence, and be influenced by, the decisions one is called upon to make in one's everyday life. These decisions will be looked at next.

Making decisions

It becomes apparent, when looking at the type of decision the childless are called upon to make, and the choices available to them in carrying out these decisions, that there are few generally valid rules. The individual personality and circumstances will determine which decisions are possible or desirable. Thus it is not easy to offer insights that are widely applicable, as it was possible to do with the discussion on coping with feelings.

However, there are a few practical suggestions which have been found helpful. Interestingly, most of these are concerned with decisions to *stop* doing certain things, because, if continued, they will make it more difficult to come to a reconciliation with oneself as a childless person. The first thing is to stop worrying about the causes of one's, and/or one's partner's, infertility. If known, it does help, but for the many who do not know, endless speculation does not make for harmony. Secondly, women who menstruate fairly regularly should make a decision to assume that their period will arrive at the end of each cycle, even if they have had intercourse during the 'fertile' days of their cycle. Those falsely raised hopes can be very damaging to morale. A third suggestion is to take care not to overburden friends by talking at length about infertility. Few friendships can tolerate high levels of stress, particularly where the relationship seems very one-sided. If you do lean heavily upon a friend in your distress, it is important that the debt be repaid where possible. The childless have a duty to listen to the problems of others in return. Although it may take courage, it does seem more sensible to take these problems to someone who has an expertise in listening and counselling. Better advice is likely to be given, and confidences are less likely to be betrayed.

Perhaps the most necessary piece of advice for some of the childless, particularly for those who know that they are infertile, rather than their partner, is to stop feeling guilty. It is hard to do this, especially if the partner responds to infertility in a hostile manner. Despite the widely held view that one partner must be 'to blame' for a couple's inability to produce a child, blame is a very inappropriate word. You have tried, maybe very hard, but been unsuccessful. You have not committed a sin, or a crime. Constant accusations from your partner or family can be very debilitating, but you should hold firm to your integrity. This may take courage and endurance. You need to show understanding towards your partner, but not to the extent of belittling yourself.

Turning to things that *ought* to be done, there are a few decisions that most of the childless will need to make. A couple may need to make a decision as to the best way to renew their sexual relationship. In many cases it is likely that harm has been done to the sexual relationship, as a result of the demands of the medical investigations. It may take time for a couple to resume a relationship that is based on the need to confirm feelings for one another, rather than a relationship dictated by the need to have sexual intercourse at certain specified times. Health factors are also important. Where one or both partners are emotionally or physically at a low ebb as a result of the stress of the fertility investigations, it may be necessary to regain health and composure first, in order to avoid placing any more stress on the sexual relationship. Fortunately, there is a more relaxed attitude to sex than there was, say, ten years ago, when there was an overemphasis on the importance of sexual performance and satisfaction in a relationship. It is easier to be human now, and patience and understanding are also considered important in the sexual relationship. But if a relationship is to survive the traumas of childlessness, and to develop beyond it, it is essential that sexual problems are not repressed, but discussed and worked at. Sexual reconciliation goes hand in hand with other aspects of the reconciliation process.[8]

When a couple have discussed together how best they can help each other to overcome their distress, and have tried to avoid apportioning blame, they need to work out a strategy for dealing with other people. How, and to whom, should they admit their infertility? It need not be assumed that it is necessary to admit this. There are some circumstances when keeping quiet on the matter is a sound policy. But in general it is helpful to the recovery of morale if the childless can discuss it when necessary without fear or embarrassment. The biggest hurdle may be informing relatives. It is likely that relatives will respond on this issue with similar measures of understanding to those they have shown in other crises within the family in the past; and in accordance with their personal feelings for the individuals concerned. Thus some of the childless will find it more difficult to cope with relatives than others. Where it is apparent that a close relative is unable to be supportive, it will be hard to bear, but it is something that has to be endured and overcome. It is made easier if the childless couple are united in their approach. Where one of them feels secretly guilty at not being able to satisfy his or her parents, it could cause a rift in the couple's relationship.

After relatives, how does one deal with friends? It may be that the problem of infertility has been compounded by seeing one's friends become pregnant and giving birth with apparent ease. Some friendships may not survive, as the one side feels they have very little in common with the other. But a few good friendships will remain, and these may need to be reconfirmed, once the childless person has come to terms with the most isolating aspects of infertility. It is important to do this if the childless are to be able to gain pleasure from their friends' delight in their children.

It is often difficult for the childless, in the early stages of their adjustment, to have too much direct contact with children. The sight of a mother holding her baby, a child playing in a garden, may trigger off feelings of terrible deprivation. Yet it is important not to feel guilty about this. Eventually, with time, it will become easier to cope with other people's children. A good friend will accept that his or her children cause difficulties for the childless, and be prepared to wait until the children seem less threatening, before the relationship is resumed with some of its old intimacy. The childless for their part, should try not to distance themselves too permanently from children. They are thereby depriving themselves of much joy. Children need the company of more than just their parents and their peer group, if they are to develop into sociable, caring adults. In thinking back over one's own childhood, it is likely that there was a special aunt or uncle who was much appreciated because he or she had time to spare, to talk and play with children. Children, despite their inexperience, may often be fairly accurate judges of the feelings and intentions of adults towards them.

The advice suggested above has been of a general nature, appropriate to the experience of many of the childless as they try to cope with their lives, and adjust to a new view of the future. Yet there may come a time when they realise that their situation does given them opportunity to adjust their lives in more fundamental ways, ways that are not open to those who have responsibilities for their children. Here it is very difficult to offer suggestions that are likely to be generally useful or appropriate. People sometimes write to the NAC office asking for advice and information on alternative lifestyles, as if there were some completely new, exciting or fulfilling way of living that was happening somewhere, that would revolutionise their lives if someone told them where to look for it. But in most cases this is not what is really wanted. The person whose idea of alternative living is to study the wild life of the Galapagos Islands, let us say, does not need to be told that he should go to the Galapagos Islands. They want advice on the way to get there and how to maintain themselves when there. Their objective is predetermined.

The childless who want to know about alternative lifestyles may not have any predetermined objectives, nor may they be particularly interested in any of the more accessible alternatives such as the radical communities and groups that consciously try to live out a different set of relationships than those that are characteristic of the nuclear family. What the childless seeking an alternative lifestyle often seem to be saying is – how can I live in present day society without feeling so bad about not having children? Is there a place for me? How can I occupy my time in more satisfying ways?

It is difficult to answer this question because it is often apparent that the people asking it already have quite full and active lives. Yet there is obviously something missing, something that fails to satisfy them in their present way of life. In some cases, maybe, what is really needed is some understanding about the meaning and purpose of what they are doing. If they could think in a more positive and outgoing way about the various activities that make up their lives, they might find that the seeds of a more satisfying life have been planted, and are growing nicely. It is in reconciling their feelings with what is happening to them that such people may find what they are looking for.

But there *are* people who seriously want, or need to consider, a very different way of living, but are not sure how to go about it, or even how to start. People can easily, through lack of experience or opportunity, become stuck in uncongenial jobs, or no job, unhappy relationships, unsatisfactory living conditions, and find themselves in a kind of mental prison. It may need both finance and courage to break out of a cycle of unhappiness and oppression. But the risk has to be taken. Most people, however gloomy their present lives, can imagine better ways of living, and it is in trying to change things, being open to new ideas, finding the courage to stand up for oneself, taking steps into the unknown, that opportunities may become apparent. The first step is always the hardest. Sometimes, there is one side of the personality that has not been given a chance to develop, that is there waiting to be released. How can you discover it? Only by being prepared to try new things, to experiment, and not necessarily in a big way. Quite small changes may lead to bigger ones, and opportunities may then present themselves that were not available before. Job, home, relationships and interests seem to be the major areas where changes could be made. If there is to be a major change in one of them, one of the others may have to be sacrificed. Nothing is without its cost. The most important thing is that the cost and potential rewards are balanced. Each of us has to find his or her mountain to climb, and his or her paradise garden to rest in.

In the long-term most of the childless will come to accept their childless situation, and find new satisfactions in their lives. They will have been strengthened by their experiences, and have become more tolerant of others. But what often takes them by surprise is that, long after they have considered themselves adjusted to their situation, some small event or experience can still affect them quite deeply, and it is as if they are back at the beginning again. The regrets and the despair threaten to overwhelm them anew. At times like this they need to know that there is nothing unusual about this feeling; it appears to be quite a common phenomenon, often related to some significant change in life experience. They also need to know that the pain will go away again, and that their adjustment to their situation is not fundamentally affected. What has been gained over the years cannot be so easily undone. Just as there have been happy times in the past, so will there be happy times in the future.

Coming full circle

Any person who emerges from a deeply disturbing experience may look back and try to analyse his or her responses to the difficulties and the darkness, and perhaps feel that he or she has failed. It seems characteristic of life that we meet and undergo experiences for which nothing in our past life has prepared us. Yet even while we struggle to understand what it is that has overwhelmed us, we may be subconsciously guided towards a way of escape, and eventually find ourselves outside, living in the world again, without being quite sure how we arrived there.

What kept us moving in the dark? Why did we not give up? According to our personality, we may see the answer as coming from within, or from without. Perhaps both. In Willy Russell's sad comedy, *Educating Rita*, there is a scene with Rita, her family and friends sitting in the pub one Saturday night, singing to the jukebox. Rita sees tears falling from her mother's eyes, and asks her why she is crying. Her mother says in reply, 'There must be better songs to sing than this'. A fragile tentative belief, that there ought to be more to life, sustains her. What she lacks is the courage to live in tune with this new, flickering awareness.

The childless may feel that it has only been their belief that they would eventually have a child of their own that has kept them going. But there are other tiny, unnamed hopes, of which the individual may be quite unaware, that give a man or woman the ability to endure adversity and extreme hardship. The human spirit has a powerful will to survive. Ronald Searle, the cartoonist, described how he, and some of his friends, survived the brutal conditions of a Japanese prisoner-of-war camp:

> Survival under those conditions was a question of attitude. You had to find something to survive *for*. There was a Dutch cavalry officer who'd escaped from Java and seen his young wife machine-gunned and drowned in a Japanese air attack – he found God. There was Duckworth, who'd coxed the Cambridge boat and who looked after everyone, organised everyone, almost took on the role of martyr. That was his therapy. My means of survival was my work. I had to survive to draw, to show the world the way it really was.[9]

It is interesting that Ronald Searle saw the will to survive as an attitude. Yet the interim solutions adopted by the prisoners were very practical. They found ways to cope with their situation that enabled them to rise above it. They expressed themselves in ways true to their nature, but these ways would also enable them to make their contribution to society in the future. Searle became an outstanding cartoonist. The Dutch officer found religion, which is a life-long commitment, and the Duckworths of this world always have a place in society. If they are not given it, they find it of their own accord.

The childless need to see themselves, and their role in society, as infinitely more complex than could be deduced just from the strength of their desire to have children. They need to ask: What is it that I possess, and am not aware of, that sustains me, and leads me to think that my life is about something more than wanting a child? Perhaps the answer is already there; waiting to be recognised, and to be understood.

13

Being childless in later life

Dear Sir or Madam,

I do not know whether I can be helped by the Association, as I am not childless due to some defect in one of us, but because we could not afford to have children, as my salary was necessary to help to support my husband's ex-wife and her two sons.

I did not see them as she was very difficult about my husband's access to the boys.

It was a terrible blow to me never to have children, even though my work as a health visitor was a great pleasure, particularly the babies.

Now my husband is dead, partly through worry over the first family and I have been retired for several years and have a brother and sister and some good friends, but I am still unhappy at having no children.

Yours truly,

This letter was received by Brenda Holliday, the Administrator of NAC. She sent an encouraging reply, describing the work of the Association, and enclosing a copy of the current newsletter. A few days later she received a second letter.

26.5.83.

Dear Mrs Holliday,

Thank you very much for your letter of May 20th. I was most interested to learn of the extent of your work helping childless couples in your journal.

As I have now reached the age of 60+ and am retired and live in a house for retired people, I do not now have contact with babies and school children as before. Friends think that living with old people, it would not be a good thing to visit elderly people.

I do some work for my church, and belong to a Gardening Club which meets every two months, I also knit garments for Oxfam. I would love to join the Association but fear I would not be able to help other childless women, as my only method is to try not to think about it, and be busy.

I would be interested to hear of other ways of living a full life. I have friends with and without families. As you say in your letter one can never get over the lack of children, but I feel there is no need to make other people miserable too.

Yours sincerely,

A small proportion of those who are childless, and among the older age groups, write to the NAC office from time to time. It is sometimes difficult to know how to advise these people, because the majority of those who write in to the Association are in the younger age groups, from 20+ to 40+. Thus the Association has much greater experience, and expertise, in dealing with the problems of those who are going through the initial stages of coming to terms with the possibility of life without children.

Yet, in writing this book, we have been made very much aware that it is important to take into account the experiences and perceptions of those who are past childbearing age, and have remained childless. We wanted to find out how their feelings about being childless have affected their later lives. When trying to decide who the older childless were, we were aware that we needed to include quite a few generations. We took the menopause, the time when a woman ceases to be capable of bearing children, as our starting point. Thus we would be including a group of people, mainly in their fifties and early sixties, many of whom would still be in paid employment. We would also be considering those who were on the verge of retirement from work, somewhere from the later fifties to the mid-sixties. We would have to decide where those who had taken early retirement, or been made redundant, fitted in. Then there were those people who were in their seventies, and finally, the 80-year-olds and above.

Unfortunately, we were unable to find much information on what it was like to be childless in any of these age groups. Within the NAC files there were comparatively few letters from older people, and there are very few members of the Association in these age groups. Even when one turns to the literature on infertility, one finds advice only for the younger couple attempting to come to terms with their situation. It is assumed (perhaps by default) that it is a once-and-for-all adjustment. Discussion on infertility and its effect in later life lies outside the scope of the topics being covered. Childlessness is very rarely mentioned or discussed in books covering middle-life and ageing. Thus, for the present chapter, we have been restricted to the small number of letters in the possession of the National Association for much of our information.

The National Committee of NAC has been aware, for some time, that the situation and feelings of the older childless are not well understood, and that the letters received from older members suggest that the effects of childlessness might well persist throughout life. The Committee has also become aware that there is a great fear among the younger members of the Association, of having to face old age without children. Those in their late thirties and early forties seem most concerned about this.

Faced with the present paucity of material on the effects of childlessness in later life, we can only offer very tentative suggestions as to how being childless is perceived and experienced, based on a very limited number of first-hand accounts. It has not been easy, first of all, to establish what kinds of treatment or solutions were suggested to people who describe their past experiences of infertility. Respondents tend to be vague: 'Babies never came. We went to see the doctor but he said we should adopt, so we gave up.'

A single woman in her sixties talked approvingly of the encouragement given to young single women to bring up their own children. 'It was not really possible in my day.' Without deep probing, it is unlikely that the trauma of the experience of discovering that they were infertile will be retrievable for these older respondents. It certainly does not come over as of any particular significance in relation to their lives as a whole. The truth may even have been distorted for social reasons:

> People don't think you've got a good marriage if kids don't come. When people mention it I just say, real sad like, we went to all the doctors, we just couldn't. They think I'm going to cry, so they cheer me up. It never occurs to them it's his fault.

The limited amount of information at our disposal does not enable us to ascertain with any confidence what it was like to discover that one was infertile in earlier periods of this century. Although it appears that in several cases adoption was not necessarily acceptable as an alternative, even when it was more generally available.

When it comes to responses to childlessness, despite the lack of sufficient first-hand accounts, it is possible to discern a pattern from the available evidence. There seem to be two possible avenues which, over time, the childless can choose to follow if they wish to mitigate the effects of childlessness. The first option is to operate within a spectrum of activities designed to cope with the time that appears to become available because one does not have responsibilities for children. The second option is to invest in people, in friendships. Both of these options satisfy certain needs, and both, conversely, have their limitations as a solution to the problems of being childless. It is possible for an individual to select both solutions. They are not mutually exclusive.[1]

Turning to the first option, the measurement of time and activities, 'filling the time' with 'activity' is seen as a device to enable one to live comfortably with oneself without too much inner turmoil.

> Childlessness, yes, well I am childless. I don't bother with that though. Its no use crying over spilt milk is it? I'm too busy for that. Your members would be well advised to keep busy rather than wallow in it.

This is some kind of compromise, a recognition that there is, or has been, some kind of problem, but the problem can, and has to be, dealt with. The woman whose letters are quoted at the beginning of this chapter copes in a similar way. She fears that she would not be much use giving advice to other childless women, because her own response is to 'try not to think about it, and be busy'. And her feeling, that 'there is no need to make other people miserable too', is not so very different from thinking that 'it's no use crying over spilt milk, is it?' Each of these statements acts as some kind of rationalisation for the response chosen.

Time, and the opportunities represented by freedom from its constraining influence, act as some kind of cultural metaphor. The childless are often told how fortunate they are to be free to do things that other people are unable to do: 'Think of all you can do now you are not tied down with babies and children. You'll be able to do more.' But is this freedom as real as others would have us believe?

> We thought we could do so much more now we had all this time. We forgot we already used the time and only wanted to change the way we used it when we wanted a baby. We found that we did not so much have to find new things to do but that we had to make the things we already did more worthwhile. It is impossible to say what difference to this a baby would have made.

'Doing more' is seen as some kind of symbol reflecting the outward manifestation of a successful life. 'Doing less' is *not* used as a measure of achievement, and is not to be recommended as a solution to free time. Relaxing, except as a temporary measure after hard work, is still thought of as some kind of 'sin' or idleness in our society. 'The devil makes work for idle hands to do' is a proverb implicitly accepted by many. We exalt the supermen and superwomen of this world who achieve forty-eight hours work in a twenty-four hour day; and many still think of the unemployed as 'idle layabouts'. The couple quoted earlier in this paragraph understood how 'time' and 'activity' fail to represent the real options presented to people. The couple initially wanted to change the way they used time, primarily because they wanted a baby; which would in consequence force them to change their habitual uses of time. A change of activity would cause changes in their use of time; however, time was always seen as of secondary importance. When they realised that they could not achieve the 'activity' they wanted (bringing up a baby), they saw that the solution could not be meaningfully represented in terms of time. The *value* of their activities became their standard of measurement. Underlying their response to their situation, and their understanding of it, is a profound wisdom, which escapes many people, as we are conditioned to believe that 'saving time' and 'using the time' are virtues.

In some cases the need for activity seems to be a stronger motivator than the need to fill time, yet the two are still implicitly linked.

> Life just went on. I expect I chose to put more into work than if I'd had a family, and that we might be a bit lonelier than others sometimes, but not by much. I know lots of mums who are lonely as hell. Much lonelier than us.

Here activity, designed to make profitable use of the time 'freed' from caring for children, and to cover the loneliness of being without children, is perceived to be not completely successful as a solution. Yet, in comparison with those who have been 'successful', in that they have had children, this childless couple do not see themselves as particularly disadvantaged.

Activity has, however, another, more powerful limitation, than just failing to combat loneliness. It is dependent, for its success in disguising isolation and in providing some kind of 'meaning' structure, on the individual's ability to fight off the effects of ageing and physical deterioration: 'I dread old age most. Till then I'll manage quite well I know. I've friends, interests and things useful to do. I just hope God takes me before I'm useless and alone.' At its most extreme, a constant emphasis on activity can make a person appear quite phrenetic to others. Such a person often seems to convey, to others who operate at a less intense level of activity, that he or she is trying to hide some inner unhappiness that would threaten to engulf him or her if it was allowed to surface. Yet this activity may often be altruistic, designed to help others, and it enables the childless to feel part of society, by being useful to others.

Activity may sometimes be related to the second option available to the childless, that of investing in friendships, or it may be replaced by it. The most positive aspect of this second response can be illustrated by reference to a widow in her late eighties, who is now living in an Old

Peoples' Home. Over the past few years three of her close friends have died; also her sister and one of her brothers. Her only visitors to the Home are her brother-in-law, and a nephew who visits once a year. When her husband was alive they both had a lot to do helping her sister with her children. The nephew who visits is 'the one I always thought was no good – but he's turned out golden to me'. This elderly lady is popular in the Home with both residents and staff, because she acts as a very cheerful influence on other residents. Because she has invested in relationships throughout her life, to help her combat childlessness, she is, in many ways, better able to cope with life in the Home than many of the women whose lives have been enclosed within the duties and obligations of their family. These others take their status in the Home from the occupations and achievements of their offspring. Yet what actually matters now is the quality of the relationships formed in the Home, rather than the lost, but longed-for relationships with the family outside the Home. This lady believes that 'people are important, and its important *here* to be a person'. Her success in making relationships is the more outstanding when one compares her with another, single person in the Home who is very much a recluse, and who antagonises both staff and residents.

Yet the woman we are concerned with does not feel that she benefits through her ability to relate to others. She feels that the staff ignore her or shout at her, because there is no-one in the outside world to stand up for her. How true this is, is difficult to say, because in comparison with others in the Home she appears to cope very well, and is active and thoughtful. To an outsider, her main problem would appear to be having such a lively mind, while at the same time having to be dependent on others for the satisfaction of many of her physical needs. But worries similar to hers are also expressed by others in different situations: 'As we have got older we've become aware we don't belong to anyone. Just no-one owes us a family duty. It isn't fair at all you know. We wanted to belong – we end up on the edge of nothing.' It would seem that 'family duty' can only be expected from very immediate relatives, probably one's children. The old lady in the Home obviously does not think that her brother-in-law and nephew come within that category of people to whom she can turn for support when she gets angry with the staff of the Home.

One problem experienced by those who are very elderly is that they may have outlived their friends. It takes time and effort to develop and maintain friendships, and by the time a childless person has passed his or her mid-eighties, they may be too frail to be able to get out to places where they might have an opportunity to socialise. Also, many old people lose confidence in their ability to cope with new relationships as they become increasingly embarrassed by their own physical deterioration. They may have problems seeing and hearing effectively; they may be more or less immobile, and incontinence may be a real handicap. Thus, they are dependent on the kindness of others for their social experiences. Yet the ability to invest in friendships probably remains a useful tool longer than the ability to be active and busy, as a means of coping with the problems of childlessness.

Where investment is made in relationships, particularly within a small, traditional community, the childless may, despite their success in relating to others, be made to feel very peripheral. A couple in their late fifties, who had very close relationships with their brothers and sisters, and all their children, and who were loved by all, still felt left out: 'With everyone else, their kids come first, even when it's clear to us that they should let them be a bit. But we can't say owt because we don't know about what it's like to have kids.' This couple felt peripheral and undervalued, even though one of their nieces had chosen to live with them after she left school. This case, like that of the lady in the Old Peoples' Home, suggests that even where people are outwardly successful in relationships, and are able to bring happiness and comfort to the lives of others, their inner feelings may not match their outward expression. Other people may never discover how the childless person really feels, or they may be completely taken aback if they ever find out.

On balance, being active in order to fill the time, and investing in friendships, remain useful responses to childlessness in later life, as long as individuals are aware of the limitations inherent in their choice of solution. But a philosophical understanding of how one fits into the pattern of life can also be a great help in coming to terms with one's situation.

> My life is many things. It is my home, my friends, my job, my inward feeling, my independence and the fact I have no children is among these things. It is sad for me and my husband. It makes me a little afraid for the future. It does not, in weighing what is important in my life, mark out the worst of my experiences. Neither has it been a springboard for freedom to do other things people used to tell me it would be. Life has gone on, bitter/sweet as it does for everybody.

The good and the bad are measured, and found to balance. There are regrets, just as there are compensations.

> Yes, I love children, and it is one of the few personal regrets that I have. They are an important influence on the way in which people grow up and develop. I think that there is a sort of continuity in the human story that requires people to have children and grow up with them, and for them to be influenced by their children.

Luckily I have had an enormous number of relationships with

children and young people. I have dozens who come to see me and ask my advice; I seem to spend my life organising their weddings, dissolving their marriages, reconciling them to their fiancés.[2]

It can be a great privilege to be allowed a place in the lives of children and young people. Being a parent is one way to take part in the human story, but a young person's life consists of much more than just a relationship with his or her parents. It *is* possible for an older childless person to have meaningful relationships with children and young people. Such relationships are not necessarily inferior to the parental relationship – their defining characteristic is that they are *different from* the parental relationship. Each type of relationship has its own value. Yet the question has to be asked how some childless people manage to make meaningful relationships with the younger generation, while others do not, for example the woman discussed at the beginning of this chapter.

The quotation in the previous paragraph was taken from an interview with Lord Goodman, on the occasion of his 70th birthday. And he is still an active man, of outstanding achievements. But there comes a time when even the alternative compensations to parenthood may cease to be available, if one lives to very late old age. In 1977, an old man of 88 wrote to the Association, in response to a radio broadcast on childlessness:

Nobody has ever called me father or grandfather. I am now alone with the memories that other people pass on to their children. I am not afraid. I am a father you see. Not to a person, but to those things I caused to be, the furniture I made, the people who relied on me. I wish you well with your Association, but never make the mistake of believing the childless are not parents. All carry that love – there are many paths to follow.

Like other older people who have contributed to this chapter by expressing their views on life without children, this 88-year-old man has been able to balance the good against the bad, and his final synthesis transcends the limitations to his everyday experiences imposed by the weakness of old age. He has an inner integrity that enables him to speak with wisdom to generations much younger than himself. Where he could so easily offer despair, in his solitude, he offers hope, and love.

These few glimpses of what it is like to be childless in later life suggest that the experience is not entirely negative, and that many of the childless will find effective ways of coping with their loss. The strength of one's inner resources seems as important as bodily strength in coping with childlessness in old age.

In the process of ageing, the meanings that an individual is able to give to the experiences of his or her life would seem to make the difference between attaining wisdom, or sinking in despair.

14

Epilogue: One woman's story

Several years ago I wrote about my experience of infertility and coming to terms with childlessness in our booklet *Unfocused Grief*. But it is less easy for me to write about those experiences now. One's perceptions change over time and with time. Peter and I have been married for 20 years now, the cat is 13, and has rheumatism in her back legs. Though she can still do a sideways double flip somersault off a hydrangea bush, if necessary, after an abortive sortie against a blue tit. Which is more than can be said of us. In twenty years of married life we have been through a great deal together. Our being together still must, I suppose, represent some kind of achievement. We ruefully say from time to time, 'We're about the longest married couple we know', as we sadly watch the break-up of yet another couple we thought were together for life.

I find difficulty in remembering much of the detail of the traumas we went through at the time of seeking infertility treatment. It was in the late 1960s, I think. Were it not for what I have already written, it is likely that many aspects of it would come as a surprise to me. As when we meet friends from the long distance past, and they remind us of something we did or said which has gone from our memory: we can now recall it but find it difficult to know why *they* remember that particular event; and *we* remember other things.

Also, when I look back and compare the treatments that were available for infertility then with what is becoming standard practice now, I am amazed. I believe I christened the hysterosalpinogram machine at our local Women's Hospital. By the time modern drug treatments, laparoscopies, donor insemination, male fertility treatments and test-tube babies had come into being, I had reconciled myself to the search for alternatives to having children. In some ways, perhaps, the choice was made easier in that these tempting miracle solutions were not dangled before me. I was also, at the time we were undergoing medical investigations, taking steps to obtain educational qualifications, which was to make it easier for me to find alternatives when our search for children failed. I had left school with A-levels, and worked until after our marriage, in jobs that gave me no satisfaction except an income. At the age of 24, with Peter's help, I changed careers. I became a temporary teaching assistant in a junior school, and then spent two years at Westhill College of Education, a very rewarding experience, and I learnt a great deal about children which has stood me in good stead over the years, and has proved very relevant to the teaching of adults. After completing my probationary teaching year in a junior school, I went to Birmingham University as a mature student, and obtained a degree at the age of 31. Since then I have gained other qualifications on a part-time basis. As a result of this, opportunities have been open to me which may not be open to those childless women who first think about alternatives when they are approaching their middle years.

There is another reason why the experience of infertility seems distant and remote, and that is that it was succeeded by a period of my life which I regarded at the time, and still do, in retrospect, as being essentially happy. A.J.P. Taylor, the historian, said of the writing of his life story:

> During most of the time when I was writing it I thought the predominant impression was one of misery – two broken marriages, each bringing great pain. Now in my changed circumstances of marital happiness I cannot understand my previous history except as an historical fact. For me it is all dead and forgotten. Happiness quickly obliterates the memories of misfortune.[1]

Likewise, it is difficult for me to invest with great emotion, from a distance, the period when we were involved in the quest for a child. Objectively seen, the period subsequent to this also had its times of unhappiness and insecurity, but the aura of those years comes over as positive and optimistic. When I first wrote about my responses to childlessness, the writing down of important experiences enabled me to detach myself from them, and to let them go.

Peter and I both had unhappy childhoods, and I think our main motivation in wanting a child was to break the chain of cause and effect. We wanted to give a child a happy home. We believed we could achieve this. I saw myself as a maternal person, rather reserved, but hiding deep feelings and capable of an intense love shared only with a few. Peter had considerable experience and understanding of young people in distress, both professionally and informally. We were, I think, in our late twenties when we thought about having a child. We did not feel strongly about having our own child, so when, after a time, I had not conceived, we enquired about adoption. We were informed that prospective adopters had to produce a doctor's letter stating that conception was not possible.

Thus we started a long series of medical investigations and tests at a women's hospital in the Midlands. It became something of a game, as we were given contradictory information, according to which doctor we saw; this was never adequate, and I used to find out what I could by reading my file upside-down from the patient's side of the doctor's table. I always seemed to have done incorrectly something I had not been told to do in the first place, and I must admit I faked some of the temperature charts. Peter was nervous because he took very little part in the tests, (men had very minor roles in infertility investigations in those days). But apart from anxiety that the doctor would forget to examine me and I would be locked in an Outpatients' cubicle overnight in a state of semi-undress, I did not expect too much. I had earlier discovered that my particular specialist did not issue letters that anyone was incapable of having children, unless she were without a womb. So I was prepared for his final indecision, when he enquired with some embarrassment how much I knew of my husband's medical history, and declined to do any further tests.

Neither was I too upset by the limited adoption prospects, because I had talked to the medical social worker at the hospital, who explained, after hearing of our family histories and Peter's medical problems, that we would be unlikely to be accepted as adopters. I have often wondered how she managed to convey this depressing information without alienating or distressing me. She must have possessed considerable professional and social skills.

The trauma came when I thought about fostering. At the time Peter was working to develop a residential community, at the Birmingham Settlement, including several adolescent boys who had never known their parents, who had been in institutions, some of them from their first week of life, abandoned and rejected. A child-care officer came to tea, so it seemed a suitable opportunity to make informal enquiries. I had my reservations while we were at the tea-table. No, she didn't like Birmingham. No, she didn't like this. Or that. She was about fifty, single, dumpy and miserable. We found a quiet room after tea. I plucked up courage, and began. I think I said something about not wanting to foster until I had finished my University course, because I would like to be at home so that I could give the child full care and attention. She said blankly, 'You don't want fostering, you want adoption. They can take the child away from you at any time. They have their own parents.' I shut up. I could not understand it. I could not see where they could take the boys at the Settlement to. They had come to us because they had no parents; no-one else wanted them. To have a child like that from a younger age would give him a much better chance in life. I later realised that the children I was thinking about were coloured, and that if I had specified that I was willing to take a non-white or older child there would have been possibilities, perhaps even for adoption. I did not realise that such categories existed, nor that adoption was primarily for babies. But by then it was too late. I resolved, after this one disastrous encounter with officialdom that, apart from consideration of the heartache involved, where children could be forcibly removed from homes where they were happy, I would never voluntarily put myself in the position of being forced to beg from public officials for whom I could have no respect.

Having rejected the idea of fostering, I was left with very little to fall back on. I found it increasingly sad every time a friend of mine became pregnant. I felt it was the end of the friendship. I also became more disillusioned with the social-work profession. Young workers often came to the Settlement to make arrangements about adolescents in care. I realised how little some of the workers knew about the youngsters in their case-load; and how poorly equipped some of them were to communicate with, or make judgments about, young people. Yet these social workers possessed considerable legal powers.

The worst period was towards the end of the time when we lived in the Settlement. I was not suited to community life. Peter always had dozens of people in need of his help; he was kept busy, under constant pressure, and consequently had little time to reflect on our situation. The lack of privacy and sleep was too much for me. I had to share Peter with far too many people (for several years after I had dreams of people walking uninvited into our house; I would shout and rave at them and tell them to get out). The only way my life was made tolerable at this time was by giving intensive remedial education to individual students in care living at the Settlement. As they improved and I began to know each student better I would come to like them and find pleasure in our encounters. A few became fond of me and I of them. I found a purpose in helping them educationally and socially, and when they left the Settlement I found my source of meaning removed, with nothing to fall back on. My only release was to talk to a very sympathetic woman doctor at the University Health Centre, who just listened, was never censorious, and was interested in the Settlement because she had done voluntary work there as a schoolgirl.

From this low point life did slowly improve. It started when I finally persuaded Peter that we had to move from the Settlement. I arranged to rent a semi-detached house, and found myself a full-time job in a technical college. These positive decisions about external matters gave me the inner confidence to begin to consider emotional factors. Peter was unhappy at the thought of being, as he saw it, forced away from what was most important to him and possessed, instead, by me. But the sense of inner release and strength I gained from living a private life and doing a job which gave me emotional satisfaction were such that, though I would not stop him from living his life (we had two homes; he could sleep at the Settlement), I would no longer take part. I can still remember walking down Selly Oak High Street that Christmas, thinking that Peter would probably have divorced me by the next Christmas, and reassuring myself that the paving-stones would still feel the same.

We eventually bought a house, and Peter slowly came to see that he could work more creatively by being more detached from the Settlement. To Peter's regret, I played a very small part in his professional life over the next few years. It is difficult to work out the rights and wrongs of this, but on balance I feel that it was a necessary stage in my emotional and intellectual development, that it had to happen before we could become closer much later on.

For me the years after I left the Settlement, and taught English as a second language in various parts of Birmingham, were very rewarding. One good thing that the Settlement had achieved for me was that I was no longer afraid of difficult people, and was able to cope with almost any bizarre classroom situation. For three years I taught newly arrived immigrants in an inner-ring junior school. It was not an easy place in which to work, but I became very attached to the staff and to the children I taught. I was sad to leave that school, but I realised that I preferred teaching adults to teaching children.

My teaching experiences taught me three things in relation to coping with childlessness. Firstly, to be fully occupied in activity, paid or voluntary, which is demanding and satisfying, leaves less time for brooding over one's losses. Secondly, over the years I made many friends, both among the staff with whom I worked, and among former students. I very gradually learnt the lesson which Peter was always trying to teach me – that of the necessity for the dispersal of affections. His point was that intense feeling directed towards one person, or a very small group, was only permissible within the family. The childless person with love and affection to give had to spread it widely, as to concentrate it would lead to disaster or failure. Any help or affection I have been able to give has, in fact, been amply rewarded. Students who have been on our courses at the University write in, sometimes years later, to tell us of their successes. The staff receive photographs and beautiful presents, and it is surprising how many former students contrive to come back on further courses. For me, all of this has led to a feeling of greater self-confidence, and a greater understanding of the varieties of social and cultural experience that make up our world. Lastly, it is important to the childless that they have achievements of their own – that they do not expect their partner alone to provide all their emotional satisfactions.

Most of my close female friends have been women I work or worked with. Two of these friendships in particular have brought me into touch with the delights of children growing up. I met Pam when we both taught at the same technical college, and from the first we became firm friends. Something I greatly missed after Pam got married and had her first baby was our weekly coffee and conversation. But Wendy was always a very special baby. She was and is very bright, and I have kept most of the drawings she did when she came to our house. Brother Patrick arrived when Wendy was three. He is now, at the delightful age of four, full of confidence and curiosity.

The two other children I have had the privilege to watch growing up have been the son and daughter of my friend Julia, whom I met when teaching in the Inner Ring. Zaffar, who was two when I first knew him, a very quiet, self-contained child, is now a handsome 11-year-old and doing well at school. Sister Roxana is very different in temperament. She was walking at 8 months, which meant she walked to the nearest mud, and put it in her mouth.

I ask myself why these children and others have given me such pleasure, when some childless women may have experienced feelings of alienation from their friends who have children. I think this is partly because I am older. I had largely reconciled myself to my condition, before I met Pam and Julia. Secondly, the friendship is with the mother, and the relationship with the children is an extension of this. As we adults put the known world to rights over a cup of tea, we re-affirm our friendship and legitimise my relationship with the children. With Zaffar and Roxana, as soon as Roxana reached the age of 5, I became 'Auntie Diane', and Peter became 'Uncle Peter'. Father had put his foot down. We had to be shown due respect. Actually, I quite like being called Auntie. But the relationship of 'Aunt' or 'Uncle' and children can only flourish with the parents' blessing. It is not so easy to develop a relationship with children where there are disagreements among the adults involved, or where the friendship with the parents fails to grow over time, possibly because the two families live far apart.

Perhaps the most important event of my late thirties was my visit to Iran. Until I was 37, the furthest I had been abroad was a day trip to Morocco on a Thompsons' holiday on the Costa del Sol. I had long wanted to go to Iran, and had slowly won Peter over to the idea, but when the opportunity came it was at such short notice that I was afraid to go. As I waved goodbye to Peter at Birmingham Airport, I thought 'This is the worst thing I have ever done'; and nearly two months later, as the plane landed at Heathrow, I thought 'This is the best thing I have ever done'.

Life was not easy in Iran; the Revolution was not far away. But the days were relatively peaceful in Shiraz, in the south, surrounded by high mountains. I taught at the University, and lived in a ramshackle old house with a shaded, walled garden, on the edge of the city.

I would get up early in my old house, and read in the shade of the garden before the sun became too hot. I remember sitting out there one morning and I suddenly said to myself, 'I am here. I am here.' The words cannot describe the experience. It was a revelation of great joy to me. A few nights later I had a memorable dream. In it I was told that I could visit India, something I had long wanted to do. Going to India was not, I think, the main theme of the dream, though I did go two years later. What the dream was telling me was that I had a future. I was not bound by the past, or restricted in the way that many people are. In that empty old house, which had purposefully been left full of dust and cobwebs by its owner, an eccentric English biologist, everything worked according to the will of nature. It was a wise house. It passed on its prescience. I sat in the garden one day and I knew that something bad would happen to me. I could not understand how my happiness could change, but I knew it would. I knew, too, that I was prepared to meet this unknown, yet known, future. (Sometime after I got back from Iran, it was discovered that I had sarcoidosis; I was very debilitated for over two years).

Before I came back to England, I had the privilege of staying with an Iranian family in Isfahan, the family of one of my students from Shiraz. I have never seen more perfect buildings than the mosques and seminaries of Isfahan. (The Taj Mahal in India is beautiful beyond description, but it lacks the reverence of the holy buildings of Isfahan). The theological college, with its rose gardens, and the elderly pilgrims queuing up for permission to make the Haj to Mecca... it was one of the most peaceful places on earth. The turquoise blue of the mosques of Isfahan fades into the blue of the sky, and when I think of Iran, I think of blue skies and swallows at sunset. The family in Isfahan still write to me. They ask me to send things out for them, and they pay me in pistachio nuts. The postman gets exhausted carrying them.

From that time on, travel became an important part of my life. Peter and I spent a marvellous Christmas in the deserts and mountains of Southern California and Nevada, and the snowbound Grand Canyon. I later went to India on my own, which was an adventure, to say the least, but I was greatly helped by some of my ex-students. India is a country impossible to assess, or come to terms with. One wonders how it all sticks together, but it does. It leaves one with a sense of amazement and bewilderment. It evokes strong responses, both negative and positive. But it has been good to meet Indian intellectuals and field workers dedicated to bringing about improvements in the lives of the poor, when it would be easy for them to ignore the situation, and to concentrate on preserving their own comforts and superior status.

When I was 40 I took up yoga, and as a result of the teachers' excellence, and practising the postures and breathing exercises, I found a new understanding of myself, and a greater sense of wellbeing. I used to call going to yoga class 'Saying hello to myself'. At the end of the initial relaxation, as we prepared to do the exercises, the teacher would say, gently, 'Be here now'. Words... but powerful thoughts. It is hard in the West to detach oneself from the trauma and pettiness of the past, and the worries and fears for the future. Just being is an achievement; wonderful to experience.

It was about this time that *New Society*, the weekly journal, started a 'children for adoption' column in its advertising section. One day I saw an advertisement asking for foster-parents for a ten year-old Pakistani boy called Nasir, who had been in a children's home for most of his life. He sounded, from the description, just the kind of boy I would enjoy looking after. I mentioned it to Peter, who was somewhat surprised, but agreed that I should go ahead. I phoned the adoption officer for Nasir's area, and the next thing I remember is the adoption officer and Nasir's social worker sitting in our front room trying to persuade us to consider fostering him with a view to adoption. They were both generous, friendly, people, and it was gratifying to feel that we seemed to meet their requirements. We were both a little unsure. Peter that, because Nasir related best to men, I might reject him; for my part, I was fearful of Nasir's coming teenage years, I didn't think I could cope with Adam and the Ants, or whoever would be top of the charts then.

I remember the end of one yoga session, with our teacher saying 'Now go home refreshed, ready to meet the demands that are made upon you'. I suddenly realised that I did have the strength to cope with Nasir. We went up North for the assessment interviews and they went well. Our names were due to come up at the next panel meeting at the end of April. About a week before this, we had a sudden phone call from the social worker. Nasir's grandmother, who had been content to leave the boy in a home for years, had suddenly had pangs of guilt and felt she should offer to adopt him. Nasir, of course, was delighted with this, she was the only family he had known. The social worker was very upset, but felt he had to go ahead with the request from grandma. We had a sympathetic letter from the adoption officer, offering to come and visit us, but we declined this. Had this happened ten years earlier we would both have been distraught. As it was, we were depressed for some weeks, and each of us individually took steps to involve ourselves in activities that would take our minds off the disappointment.

I ask myself why we came through this experience relatively unscathed. There are several possible reasons. The first is that both of us sensed that to foster Nasir we would have to sacrifice quite a few things in our lives that we found worthwhile. Thus he was not filling a hole in our lives. Secondly – for me the most important reason – I was using Nasir as a test of the direction in which my life should go. When the answer was 'no', it was quite clear to me that our lives were not meant to be about the bringing up of children. Our duty lay towards the wider world. Thirdly, to have been accepted by the social workers as suitable to foster and adopt was a confirmation that we were valued, and that we measured up to a demanding standard. It was, in a way, good for our self-confidence.

People sometimes ask whether coming to terms with childlessness makes one a better, more sympathetic person. In my case it made me a *different* person, but it is suffering over a long period from the after-effects of an illness contracted while abroad that has made me aware of the need to be more compassionate. It has led me to question several of the values that I once took for granted, and I feel very much as if I have reached the end of one stage of my life, and am about to enter another, but the way ahead is not always clear. Sometimes the only certainty has been the constancy of Peter's love, and the knowledge that our friends care for us. Strangely, in entering the realms of the walking wounded, I feel as if I have joined the mass of the human race. I have become aware that, in the balance of give and take over the past few years, I have had a very good bargain. I received much more than I gave. Now happiness seems less important than trying to understand. Now the giving has to become less conditional.

This chapter is one account of childlessness. And here I meet with problems. It is difficult to find a direct relationship between what is happening to me now, and the effects of childlessness. What I am experiencing now makes more sense to me as an account of entering middle age, which it is. I ask myself whether there are any significant social stages that people with children would be going through in the early forties, and find that our present society admits of so much variety that there is nothing here to latch on to. Many of our friends married fairly late and still have pre-teenage children. Others married early, and their children are independent, but the children are not getting married. At a recent wedding, the groom was 34, and his parents in their mid-sixties. It is all very confusing.

There may be ages or stages in one's life when being childless is more distressing than at other times. The twenties and early thirties seem to be more difficult ages for most of the childless. There is an element of competition among younger people that can be very cruel to those unable to compete. The media exploit this – just look at the advertisement for suntan lotion. The girl with the better tan (because she has used the 'right' product) is off-hand and rude to her pale friend. She does not offer to share the sun-tan lotion with her. Such advertisements play on the insecurities of young people; and it is possible that younger women with babies and young children do express their pride in ways that are hurtful to the childless, even if they do not intend any hurt. But by their forties most people, whether they have children or not, have become aware of their mortality. They have had sufficient common experience to be aware that as individuals they are expendable, and, particularly in a time of recession, they may have had to settle for second best. The days when they were considered 'promising' are very finally over. Most have done as well as they ever will in their careers or jobs (unless they are MPs or world leaders)!

For those with older children, there is also the realisation that as they themselves are ageing, and slowly deteriorating physically, their children are coming into their own and taking over. Though there is pride in watching one's children succeed, the teen years are often a time of tension and stress for parents. And for some, children may have been so central to their lives, that when they leave home the parents go through a form of grief (the 'empty nest' syndrome). Beyond this, it is difficult to discern a pattern for the forties.

Socially, then, it is difficult to decide where Peter and I belong as a childless couple. We are very fortunate in that we live amongst very tolerant people. Our friends come from a wide variety of social backgrounds, and include people both younger and older than ourselves who never make us feel excluded. But this might not be true if we lived in a different type of community, such as a suburban housing estate composed mainly of families with young children; or an isolated village where everyone knows what everyone else is doing better than they know themselves.

The society within which the childless live may or may not make it more difficult for them to be accepted. But childlessness is also a personal matter, and I ask myself whether there are any personal problems uniquely experienced by the childless. Before attempting to answer this, I feel that it is important to see how the experience of infertility relates to an individual's general life experience. The different types of life experience are likely to have an effect on the way the problems of the childless are perceived. There are, as I see it, three main categories of relationship. The first, possibly the most common category, is where infertility is experienced by an individual whose life has generally been satisfying. Such a person has had good relationships with his or her parents, and childhood is remembered as a generally happy time. This kind of person is fairly well equipped to deal with problems of adult life, and infertility comes as a major shock, because the failure to produce children is so out of step with the person's beliefs about the natural progression of life. The second kind of person also experiences infertility as a major shock; but his or her responses are complicated by earlier experiences of failure in relationships and events. Into this category come those who have experienced unhappy relation-ships with parents, or lack of success in school, severe illness, or a variety of complicating factors which are known to lead to a poor sense of self-esteem. Infertility is the most debilitating experience among many negative ones. The third kind of relationship is where the negative features of early life are present, as in the second description, and infertility is experienced; but in the sum of things it is not in retrospect considered the worst experience among the many bad ones. This latter reflects my own view of my experiences.

Yet I can perceive difficulties that the childless are especially likely to experience, though the problems are not unique to the childless. The first is the fear of the death of one's partner. This sometimes comes over me – the terrible emptiness and loss of meaning I would have to endure if Peter died. When I am feeling strong, one half of me says that I would cope. The other half says that the light would go out of my life. Although I am aware that bereavement is feared by many people in circumstances different from mine. The soldier's wife may live with a kind of fear very akin to that experienced by the childless. Elaine Evans, interviewed on television about her feelings since her husband's death in the Falklands, said 'I often thought if Ken were to suddenly appear I'd give him a kick to express how I felt about being left on my own.'[2] That she has two young children does not make the loss any easier to bear.

The second problem experienced by the childless is that as they get older or become ill and less independent, there is no one from whom they can of right demand help. They have to earn this help from friends or neighbours by living in such a way that others feel it worth their while to help them; or feel some sense of duty because of favours done to them by the childless person in the past. It is a dreadful experience to lie in bed sick and alone, saying 'God, please help me', and to know that there are about a million people living in the same city as oneself, and not to be able to ask for help without feeling one is taking up another's time unnecessarily, or even that it is wrong to put oneself under an obligation to those outside the family. Only the family have to accept us as we are. The childless may suffer great isolation in times of stress, and it is, I feel, some inadequacy in our conception of society, that we feel we can only expect help from close relatives; we fail to see that most people have fewer relatives then families had in the past, or that many families now live further apart. We have failed to make alternative social arrangements for mutual help and caring in time of need. We can expect the state to provide the structure for caring, but it is people who have to do the actual caring; not only because they are paid to do it, but because they care. We seem to have reached an impasse where the elderly are frightened to go into Homes, which they regard as updated versions of the Workhouse. Yet the stresses and strains of caring for the elderly are such that very few individuals are able to undertake this task for any length of time without sacrificing their own wellbeing.

The third problem that may be experienced by the childless is that in their attempts to compensate for their lack of a family, they become so active in their work or leisure, or both, that they leave themselves very little time to come to themselves, or to reflect on their situation. The result is that when they are brought to a halt, by exhaustion or circumstance, they experience a painful emptiness until their bodies and minds wind down to a rate more in keeping with their natural metabolism. This experience is not restricted to the childless. It is almost a disease of the Western world. It is a very common avoidance response to unwelcome or distressing thoughts. Superficially it represents a way out of mental difficulty, but it stores up trouble in the long term. The childless do have to stop from time to time and ask themselves, in view of their circumstances, which are slightly different from those who have responsibility for children, whether the life they are leading offers a really meaningful alternative.

Are there any solutions to these problems? I doubt whether they are completely soluble. But there are partial solutions. It is important that the childless attempt to make friendships over a wide range of age groups, and with people of diverse backgrounds and experience. Despite any appearance they may give, many people are not entirely fulfilled by family life, particularly as they grow older. Most people do in fact have room in their lives for friendships with those who may appear different from them. With experience, people generally become more tolerant and recognise a mutual need for friendship. Even those with children know that under our present social arrangements, if they live long enough, their final days are just as likely to be spent among strangers as among family. Both those with children and those without recognise a common fear of loneliness in later life. Those few whose children will give them love, care and freedom in their old age are fortunate indeed. The rest of us must cling together for support.

There are two things which often inhibit the childless from making friendships. One is that not everyone is naturally gregarious. Some need more solitude than others. Some possess the necessary skills for friendship, while others feel awkward and lacking in confidence. For the introverted soul it may be difficult to make the extension needed if one is to gain friends. But social skills can be learnt, and self-confidence gradually comes with experience. And with time the childless can come to share in the joys and achievements of others, particularly their children.

The second inhibition affecting the childless is that they see themselves beset by a set of unique problems that separate them from others. Many people with a serious problem think of themselves as unique. Yet life throws up difficulties for most at some time or another. All people suffer – in different ways – but they suffer. It is a measure of our common humanity. And it is in understanding this, and in taking an imaginative leap beyond ourselves, in giving to others, that we receive comfort in return.

Notes

Chapter One

1 In view of the continued growth of NAC over the years, and the development of administrative problems connected with the increase in size of NAC, Geoffrey Allen was invited to act as consultant. He carried out a review of NAC and made certain recommendations for its future development (*National Association of the Childless: Review*, October, 1985). He saw the priorities for the Association as follows (in descending order of importance):

   1. Maintenance of a public image
   2. Promotion of the cause of childless persons
   3. Provision of information
   4. Provision of counselling and support

   He considered that the central office should be mainly concerned with the policy-making aspects; that the regional committees and contacts should be mainly concerned with the counselling; and that a Field Officer should be appointed to act as someone in the middle, linking the centre and the regions. The report was accepted in principle by the NAC Committee, and ways of implementing the recommendations are under consideration. However, the NAC Committee felt that NAC now needed a fulltime Director rather than a Field Officer and it is for this post that funds are being sought.

2 The most useful books covering the medical aspects of infertility are listed in the selected reading section at the end of this book. *The Experience of Infertility* by Naomi Pfeffer and Anne Woollett, Virago, 1983, gives a useful annotated list of most of the simplified medical accounts of infertility that have been published in this country. The notes to Chapter Two of their book discuss the presentation of infertility in medical textbooks.

3 Discussion of the available statistics on the extent of infertility is to be found in Chapter 2, 'Who are the Childless?', particularly pp. 17–20.

Chapter Two

1 Elaine Campbell has carried out an interesting study of the motivations of a selected group of couples who decided to remain childfree. *The Childless Marriage: An Exploratory Study of Couples Who Do Not Want Children*, Tavistock Publications, 1985.

2 See *The Artificial Family: A Consideration of Artificial Insemination by Donor*, by R. Snowden and G. D. Mitchell, Unwin Paperbacks, 1983. Chapter 2, on the donor insemination couple, goes into some detail on the reasons why donor insemination may be preferred to adoption. Though it would seem that the popularity of donor insemination is in many ways related to the decline of adoption as a feasible solution to childlessness, those who choose donor insemination may feel that it is less risky from the genetic point of view. At least 50 per cent of the donor insemination child's genetic inheritance is known, which is not the case with adoption.

3 The figure of 15 per cent is given by the following:
   B. Eck Menning, *Infertility: A Guide for the Childless Couple*, Prentice-Hall, 1977.
   E. Philipp, *Childlessness: Its Causes & What to Do About Them*, Hamlyn Paperbacks, 1984.

J. J. Stangel, *Fertility & Conception: An Essential Guide for Childless Couples*, Paddington Press, 1979.

A. Stanway, *Why Us? A Common-sense Guide for the Childless*, Thorsons, 1984.

Eck Menning and Stangel are both writing for an American audience. Although both of these books contain bibliographies, the figure of 15 per cent is not related to any one source. Philipp and Stanway, writing in a UK context, do not provide a bibliography, or give sources for their figure of 15 per cent.

4   Stanway, *op. cit.*, p. 12 states that there have been many surveys of primary infertility, and that figures of between 11 per cent and 22 per cent have been quoted. Yet he does not give any sources for these surveys.

R. Newill, *Infertile Marriage*, Penguin, 1974, gives the figure of 10 per cent.

Garrey *et al.*, *Gynaecology Illustrated*, Longman, 1978, uses the same figure; and so does P. Saunders, *Womanwise: Every Woman's Guide to Gynaecology*, Pan, 1981.

5   Stangel, *op cit.* These figures appear in an Appendix, and are not related to a particular source.

M. P. Vessey *et al.*, 'Fertility after stopping different methods of conception', *British Medical Journal*, i (1978), pp. 265–7, calculate a pregnancy rate of 64 per cent after three months exposure to pregnancy. After twelve months this rate rises to 90 per cent, and after two years to 95 per cent. I. D. Cooke *et al.*, discuss these and other relevant statistics, and reach the following conclusion: 'Assuming normal cohabitation and no coital problems, it is easy to see that, in the UK ... 95 per cent of the population should have achieved a pregnancy after two years exposure.' They suggest that a reasonable suspicion of infertility should be entertained after twelve months exposure (see Cooke *et al.*, 'Fertility and infertility statistics: their importance and application', *Clinics in Obstetrics & Gynaecology*, vol. 8, no. 3 (Dec 1981), p. 532).

6   M. G. R. Hull *et al.*, 'Population study of causes, treatment & outcome of infertility', *British Medical Journal*, 291, 14 December 1985, pp. 1693–7.

7   Philipp, *op cit.*, pp. 13–14.

8   Philipp & Carruthers, eds., *Infertility*, Heinemann, 1981.

9   See Eck Menning, *op. cit.*, pp. 5–6, and Stanway, *op. cit.*, pp. 12–13.

10 *The Demographic Yearbook* published annually by the United Nations in New York gives details of estimates of mid-year populations by country. The statistics for 1981 and 1982, in particular, suggest a trend towards zero population growth in certain countries. The figures shown include the estimates for the previous nine years. Some caution is needed, however, in interpreting the UN figures. The population figures given by the UN for the UK in relation to live births were higher than those provided by the UK Office of Population Censuses and Surveys. For 1980, the UN figure is 752,423, and the OPCS figure is 656,234. This suggests that the UN may be underestimating the size of the falling trend in some populations.

The Political Economy of Demographic Change, by John Ermisch, Heinemann Educational Books/Policy Studies Institute, 1983, describes the possible causes and effects of the present UK trend towards a falling population. Ermisch's theory is that the fall in the birth-rate is related to rises in the level of women's wages, making women reluctant to stop work to have children. The longer women postpone childbearing, the smaller will be the size of their family. Ermisch spells out the difficulties of supporting an ageing population, with only two workers to every pensioner by the year 2030.

Chapter Three

1   See the selected reading list on page 181. Also, Pfeffer and Woollett, *op. cit.*, contains a useful annotated summary of most of the available books on infertility for the non-specialist.

2   This point has been made by Dr Jack Glatt, medical adviser to the National Association for the Childless; and the view is supported by several gynaecologists. It arises mainly from the belief that unexplained infertility is primarily a problem of diagnosis; and that a more widespread, thorough and imaginative use of the laparoscope, particularly at the time of ovulation, would reveal problems more readily. These problems might then be more easily treatable. There has, however, been no research to corroborate this.

3   See Overstreet *et al.*, 'Penetration of human spermatozoa into the human zona pellucida and the zona-free hamster egg: a study of fertile donors and infertile patients', *Fertility and Sterility*, 33(1980), pp. 534–42.

4   See Stanway, *op. cit.*, pp. 66–7. He describes Swedish research on the T-mycoplasma infection, but does not provide a source for this. The infection is also mentioned in Eck Menning, *op. cit.*, p. 26.

5   This is a rather fraught area of infertility diagnosis and treatment. The medical understanding of psychosexual factors in infertility seems to be that the factors can be both a cause and an effect of infertility. A certain percentage of infertility cases will be men or women who are unable to consummate intercourse. E. E. Philipp and G. B. Carruthers, *op. cit.*, suggest that between 5 and 10 per cent of couples will have this problem, and that the causes are *not* always psychogenic (i.e., caused by the mind). Garrey *et. al.*, *Gynaecology Illustrated*, supports this position. However, where a male specialist is dealing with a female psychosexual problem which the individual specialist believes to be psychogenic, there may be antagonism on both sides. The description and explanation of vaginismus in Newill, *op. cit.*, relates to a view of a female motivation which would not be accepted by feminists, and might also alarm many other women, and men! Pfeffer and Woollett, *op. cit.*, Chapter 4, discuss the problems of deciding whether a psychosexual problem is the cause or result of infertility. In their notes to the chapter, they give a variety of references supporting their arguments. Stanway, *op. cit.*, and Eck Menning, *op. cit.*, discuss the sexual problems that can arise as a result of the stresses of infertility investigations. In this present book the myths about childlessness as being primarily the result of a sexual disorder are discussed in chapter four.

6   This would appear to be a controversial area. Stanway, *op. cit.*, suggests that women's fertility might be affected by stress, which causes the higher centres of the brain to turn off the ovulation-stimulating hormones. In Chapter 6 he deals with the difficulties of separating the mental and physical causes of infertility, and suggests that treatment should take into account the whole person. Newill, *op. cit.*, p. 157 suggests that sperm production by men might be affected by stress, as a result of reduction in production of the gonadotrophic hormones. He also suggests that anxiety can cause the thyroid to overact. Eck Menning quotes Swedish research showing that city dwellers had lower fertility rates than those who lived in rural areas (*op. cit.*, 49–50). However, the relationship of stress to infertility remains speculative, and it has to be borne in mind that fertility investigations are often, of themselves, stressful experiences. Philipp and Carruthers *op. cit.*, p. 5, recognise this, and they try to alleviate stress by running their fertility clinic on a very personal basis. 'Female treatments', a paper by Barbara Mostyn, Chairperson of the National Association for the Childless, describes the stress experienced by women undergoing fertility investigations. This paper formed the introduction of the NAC evidence submitted to the Warnock Inquiry in 1983.

Chapter Four

1   M. Warnock, *A Question of Life: The Warnock Report on Human Fertilisation and Embryology*, Basil Blackwell, 1985.

2   See 'Artificial insemination by donor: a report of attitudes of members of the

National Association for the Childless', by D. J. Owens, Dept. of Sociology, University College, Cardiff. A version of the report was presented to the Warnock Inquiry for its report to the Government on human fertilisation and embryology. (See also note 29 below.)

3 The problem of secrecy in relation to the present legal status of AID is dealt with in: Owens, *op. cit.*; Snowden, Mitchell, *op. cit.*; Warnock, *op. cit.*

R. and E. Snowden devote a chapter to the issue in their *Gift of a Child*, George Allen & Unwin, 1984. The legal aspects are covered in D. C. Parker, 'Legal aspects of artificial insemination and embryo transfer', *Family Law*, vol. 3, ch. 6, 1980, pp. 103–7.

The effect on children of discovering that they were conceived by AID is graphically described in two newspaper articles: (a) John Cunningham, 'When father is a missing link', *The Guardian*, 2.11.83. The experience of Candy Turner, conceived by AID, led her to form an organisation called Donor's Offspring. (b) Christopher Ree, *The Guardian* 31.7.84, described the experience of a girl conceived by AID and born into a Jewish family who was physically very different from the rest of her family and who later traced the donor, to discover that he was probably the Irish Catholic doctor who had made the AID arrangements and who had promised her parents a Jewish donor.

4 The ordering of these topics reflects the order in which they are dealt with in Warnock, *op. cit.*

Other works which deal with these issues include: L. B. Andrews, *New Conceptions*, St Martin's Press, 1984; J. Harris, *The Value of Life*, Routledge & Kegan Paul, 1985; P. Singer and D. Wells, *The Reproductive Revolution: New Ways of Making Babies*, Oxford University Press, 1984. Andrews relates mainly to the American context, and Singer and Deane emphasise the Australian position.

5 Discussed in Harris, *op. cit.*; Singer and Wells, *op. cit.*; Warnock, *op. cit.* (see note 1).

6 Figures for success rates were given by Patrick Steptoe, in *The Society, Science and Sex Debates: Made in a Lab*, A Granada film broadcast on Channel 4 television in 1986.

Woman's age	No. of embryos replaced	Chances of pregnancy
Under 35	3	35–40%
Nearer 40	fewer than 3	less than 20%

For other IVF practitioners, the figures for 1984 in note 8 (see below) are probably the most recent ones available. However, Professor Ian Craft (personal communication) suggests that the more recent IVF experience shows a general improvement, with perhaps an average 30 per cent success rate.

7 The first public announcement that the GIFT technique had been used appeared in a *Sunday Times* article, 31.3.85, by Tony Osman, 'A gift for the childless'. Attention was drawn to the imminent birth of a child in Texas using a technique developed by Ricardo Asch of the University of Texas.

Ian Craft, Director of Gynaecology at the Cromwell Hospital, London, currently practises this technique in appropriate cases.

8 Gynaecologists recognise that complications are more likely in multiple pregnancies, that there is a greater risk of prematurity, and some uncertainty about the long-term prognosis of the babies born. Dr Patrick Steptoe and his team at Bourn Hall, Cambridgeshire, will only replace a maximum of three embryos. Other specialists feel that the major area of risk and choice is between having one or more babies, and having no baby at all; and so prefer to use their discretion as to the number of embryos replaced in any one case, thus slightly increasing the risk of a multiple pregnancy. Professor Ian Craft produced the following figures in 1984 ('Remember the childless', *The Times*, 22.6.84):

Combined results from nine clinics showing pregnancy rate following embryo transfer

Number of embryos transferred	Number of patients	Number of pregnancies (%)
1	1317	172 (13.05)
2	766	188 (24.5)
3	347	87 (25.07)
4	141	46 (32.6)
5	43	11 (25.6)
6	18	8 (44.4)
Total	2632	512 (19.5)

As the success rates for IVF rise, it will be easier for doctors to implant fewer embryos with greater confidence in a successful outcome.

9   There was controversy in the media when a 31-year-old woman gave birth to quadruplets in May 1984, as a result of IVF. She had three children by her first husband, had been sterilised ten years earlier after a baby died, and her marriage broke up. She remarried and separated, and the IVF quads were from her relationship with another man.

However, at the other end of the spectrum it has been argued by some feminists that 'in a technologically advanced society the unavailability ... of test-tube conception may be seen as constraints on women's reproductive freedom' (A.M. Jaggar, *Feminist Politics and Human Nature*, Harvester Press, 1983, p. 319).

10   The newspaper reports of this event are very confusing. *The Guardian*, 13.1.84, heads theirs 'Baby is born from donated egg', but proceeds to talk about prenatal adoption (which is relevant to *embryo* donation). The programme under which the baby was born was the embryo donation programme at Queen Victoria Medical Centre, Monash University, Melbourne, Australia. It becomes clear when reading a short report by the team in Letters to Nature (*Nature*, 307, 12.1.84, p. 174), that embryo donation is a generic term used to cover both egg and embryo donation, which Warnock *op. cit.*, treats separately. The report, by P. Lintjen, A. Trounson, J. Leeton, J. Findlay, C. Wood and P. Renon is titled 'The establishment and maintenance of pregnancy using in vitro fertilisation and embryo donation in a patient with primary ovarian failure'. Yet the sperm fertilised was that of the recipient's husband, not of a donor – 'using procedures described previously for embryo donation, a single oocyte was inseminated with spermatozoa prepared from a semen sample from the recipient's husband'.

Singer and Wells, *op. cit.*, p. 79 write as if they are dealing with embryo donation rather than egg donation.

11   Warnock, *op. cit.*, Ch. 6

12   Harris, *op. cit.*, p. 113, refers to 'prenatal adoption', a term he takes from R.G. Edwards and J. Purdy (eds), *Human Conception in vitro*, Academic Press, 1981, p. 360. Warnock, *op. cit.*, p. 40; Harris sees it as having an advantage over normal adoption in that the couple share the experience of pregnancy and childbirth and mother and child experience bonding during pregnancy. (Warnock is against one particular technique used in embryo donation (lavage), as it may be harmful to the egg donor.) Singer and Wells, *op. cit.*, p. 80, see embryo donation as an acceptable extension of IVF, as the effects on the child can be no worse than those experienced by an adopted child, or child by AID, on learning the true facts of his/her origins.

13   Warnock, *op. cit.*, p. 40.

14   Singer and Wells, *op. cit.*, pp. 110–11, make use of these terms.

15   See Warnock, *op. cit.*, Ch. 8.

16 Commercial surrogacy is permitted in several states in the USA. Details of existing surrogate mother programmes are given in Andrews, *op. cit.*, pp. 317–18. Commercial surrogacy arrangements are illegal in the UK (see note 21 below).

17 This was mentioned by Noel Keane (who runs a surrogacy programme in Michigan, USA) as his experience on the Channel 4 Television *Society, Science and Sex debates: Cash on Delivery*, broadcast in 1986. Keane's experiences in the surrogacy field are described in N. Keane and D. Breo, *The Surrogate Mother*, Everest House, 1981, where he refers to the unenforceable nature of contracts on p. 234. Some of the stories of couples who make use of surrogates are rather distressing. The area is a legal, financial and emotional 'minefield'.

18 These issues are raised by several participants in the *Society, Science and Sex debates: Cash on Delivery* broadcast (see note 17).

19 This scenario forms the plot of a novel by Gwynneth Branfoot, *The Wife Wants a Child*, Methuen, 1983. Also, the novel by Deborah Moggach, *To Have and to Hold*, Penguin Books, 1986.

20 Singer and Wells, *op. cit.*, pp. 128–30 see full surrogacy as psychologically much less harmful for all the parties involved, parents, surrogate and child. Its acceptance would mean fewer partial surrogacies.

21 Under the Surrogacy Arrangements Act, 1985, the following are forbidden on a commercial basis:
   (a) initiating or taking part in negotiations with a view to making a surrogacy arrangement;
   (b) offering or agreeing to negotiate the making of such an arrangement;
   (c) compiling information with a view to its use in making or negotiating the making of such an arrangement.
   It is also illegal to advertise any aspect of such an arrangement.

22 A baby was born in March, 1984, in Melbourne, Australia, after her embryo was frozen. Her mother had eleven eggs removed for IVF, three were immediately implanted, and six of the remaining eggs frozen. The first IVF operation failed, and the six eggs were taken out of storage. Four were damaged, the other two were implanted, and one survived. The medical team that were responsible for this were headed by Professor Carl Wood, and the freezing technique was developed by Dr Alan Trounson (see report in the *Sunday Times Magazine*, 13.5.84, 'A frozen miracle called Zoe').

23 A case under current discussion is that of a couple, where the husband wrote a note shortly before he died of cancer, requesting that his deep-frozen sperm be used to inseminate his childless wife. The wife was being treated for possible *in-vitro* fertilisation, and her consultant referred the case to the hospital ethics committee, who decided that the wife could have her husband's sperm, but the hospital would not treat her. The issues involved in this case are extremely complex, in the absence of any law which specifically governs such a case. (See 'Is there life after death?' by Andrew Veitch, *The Guardian*, 25.9.85.)

24 Warnock, *op. cit.*, Ch. 11, divides research into two categories: pure research aimed at increasing and developing knowledge of the very early stages of the human embryo; and applied research, which is research with direct diagnostic or the therapeutic aims for the human embryo, or for the alleviation of infertility in general. It does not include new and untried treatments undertaken to alleviate the infertility of a particular patient.

25 Warnock, *op. cit.*, Ch. 12, suggests a list of (mainly future) techniques that would require controls: trans-species fertilisation; use of human embryos for drug testing; ectogenesis; gestation of human embryos in other species; parthenogenesis; cloning; embryonic biopsy; nucleus substitution; prevention of genetic defects. The techniques are also discussed in Harris, *op. cit.*, Ch. 7, and Singer and Wells, *op. cit.*, Chs 5–7.

26   The quarterly newsletter, *Ethics and Medicine: A Christian Perspective*, published by Rutherford House, Edinburgh, presents a viewpoint which is generally against embryo research for religious and ethical reasons. The article by Isobel Grigor, 'Responses to Warnock: a review', (vol. 2:2, 1986, pp. 25–7, 31) presents the responses of the different churches to the Warnock Report.

Some members of the Warnock Committee did not feel they could assent to the majority recommendations on embryo research (see 'Expressions of Dissent A & B', pp. 90–4). The Unborn Child (Protection) Bill was originally presented to Parliament by the Right Hon. Enoch Powell in 1984–5, but was 'talked out' in the Commons. The most recent version of the Bill, no. 28/1985–6 was presented on 4.12.85 by Ken Hargreaves, but was again 'talked out'. The Bill would have prevented any human embryo being created, kept or used for any other purpose than enabling a child to be borne by a specified woman. It is likely that a further attempt will be made to introduce a Private Members Bill of this kind in the 1986–7 session. This shows the strength of feeling that exists on both sides over this issue.

27   It is difficult to know exactly when an embryo (or foetus) becomes capable of experiencing pain. Warnock, *op. cit.*, p. 65, distinguishes between the identification of the beginnings of the central nervous system, and the beginnings of functional activity. The former is given as 2–23 days after fertilisation, the latter is 'thought to be considerably later'. (The Report quotes the Royal College of Obstetricians and Gynaeocologists suggestion of seventeen days as the point when early neural development begins). Singer and Wells, *op. cit.*, p. 97, refer to the central nervous system beginning to form at six weeks, but are unclear as to when consciousness begins. Harris, *op. cit.*, p. 118, suggests the embryo may possibly not feel pain for as long as up to eighteen weeks.

28   Warnock, *op. cit.*, p. 66.

29   In Written Answers to Questions in the House of Commons on 25 July 1986, Sir John Osborn asked what main areas dealt with in the Warnock report were now considered suitable for legislation, and whether a Green or White Paper would be published indicating the options before presenting the legislation to Parliament.

Mr Barney Hayhoe (Minister of State for Social Services) referred him to a Written Answer to Questions, no. 14, 25 March 1986, given to Mr Alton:

> The Government are aware of the strongly held views of many honourable members about this issue [embryo experimentation]. As my predecessor and I have indicated to the House, the Government intend to introduce legislation on this and other matters dealt with in the Warnock Report on human fertilisation and embryology as soon as practicable.

30   A members' survey was recently carried out by the National Association of the Childless on the subject of infertility treatment controversies. The results of the questionnaire are in the process of being analysed. The questionnaires answered by male members showed strong support for the Warnock Report, including support for IVF and donor insemination (AID). The need for counselling for people considering these treatments was also supported. There was strong opposition to commercial surrogacy, but opinion was divided as to whether non-commercial surrogacy should be permitted. There was no clear pattern to the answers given to questions about the acceptability of various 'futuristic' treatments. Many were unsure, or failed to answer these questions.

One area where male members disagreed with Warnock was over the need for secrecy as regards the origins of children conceived by artificial insemination by donor. Warnock is against secrecy, but the NAC members surveyed were strongly in favour of maintaining secrecy. It would seem that members of NAC who live in small rural communities are more worried about a possible stigma being attached to their child if his/her origins were known – but this is something that needs further research.

The women's responses are in the process of being analysed. Results so far appear to be in broad agreement with those of the men's questionnaires. (See also note 2 above.)

Chapter Five

1 As was suggested in notes 5 and 6 of Chapter Three, psychological aspects of infertility are not easy to interpret or explain, and it is not always easy to ascertain whether psychological problems are causing infertility, or vice-versa. The problems may be exacerbated because the gynaecologist is not an expert on human behaviour (see Garrey *et al.*, op. cit. p. 402); and conversely, those with psychiatric training may not be experts in fertility.

2 We are grateful to Barbara Eck Menning, for first making us aware of the existence of the common myths about childlessness.

3 See *The Provision, Use & Evaluation of Medical Services for the Subfertile: an analysis based on the experiences of Involuntarily Childless Couples*, by David J. Owens and Martin W. Read, S. R. U. Working Paper No. 4, University College, Cardiff, 1979.

4 See Owens and Read, *op. cit.* They refer to Newill, *op. cit.* and Stangel, *op. cit.* Stanway, *op. cit.*, gives the same figure. Pfeffer and Woollett, *op. cit.*, arrive at the figure of 35 per cent through a survey of the available literature.

5 Philipp and Carruthers, *op. cit.*, p. 5.

6 *Ibid.* pp. 18–20.

7 This point has been made by Stanway, *op. cit.*, p. 43 and Philipp, op. cit., pp. 60–1. Lucienne Lanson, *From Woman to Woman*, Penguin, 1983, pp. 27–8, suggests that couples need to have sexual intercourse 3–4 times a week, and that less frequent intercourse will increase the amount of time it takes for a woman to conceive. There does not appear to be any research which proves this, however.

8 The compact edition of the *Oxford English Dictionary*, 1971, includes under its meaning 2a, both the power of procreation and the capacity for sexual intercourse. The Collins *English Dictionary*, Chambers *Twentieth Century Dictionary*, and Longman's *New Universal Dictionary* also include procreative power within the meaning of the terms 'virile' or 'virility'. However, medical usage distinguishes between impotence and infertility, and most textbooks dealing with the subject of male fertility stress the need to reassure an infertile man that the two conditions are unlikely to be connected with each other (see Philipp and Carruthers, *op. cit.*, and Garrey *et al.*, op. cit.; also The *Penguin Medical Encyclopaedia* by Peter Wingate, Penguin, 1976).

9 Michael Todaro, *Economic Development in the Third World*, Longman, 1981, gives a variety of statistics relevant to world population estimates. In Chapter 6, 'The population debate', he shows that, in 1980, more than two-thirds of the world's total population lived in developing countries, and less than one-third in the economically developed nations. In developing countries, children under the age of 15 form almost half the population. In developed countries, children under 15 account for a quarter of the population. Thus we can work out the percentage of the world's children under 15 who live in countries characterised by poverty, inequality and low productivity.

	developing nations, %	economically developed nations, %
Distribution of population	70	30
Children under 15 as a percentage of world population	35	7½

This gives us the ratio of about 4:1 for the numbers of children in developing nations, compared to those in the developed nations. Thus, about 80 per cent of the world's children live in developing countries, and about 20 per cent in the developed nations. These figures do not imply that all children in developing countries will suffer because of a lack of provision for basic life-sustaining needs, or that all children in the economically developed countries will be born into families that have the means to provide for them adequately. Statistics which are used as indicators of poverty or affluence will show some kind of cline, with very poor nations at one end, and the richer countries at the other end, and differences within the countries. In terms of resource use, for example, the 30 per cent of developed nations consume 80 per cent of the world's resources, leaving 20 per cent of the resources for the other 70 per cent of the population. (The United States alone, accounting for 6 per cent of the world's population, utilises 40 per cent of world resources).

N.B. The figures given in the 3rd edition (1985) suggest that the gap between developed and developing countries has continued to widen, with over 75 per cent of world population living in the developing countries (p. 183).

10 Richard Slaughter, in his paper 'Futures education: Why we need to teach for tomorrow', draws a future web based on possible consequences of doubling the human life-span. Three immediate effects are – more elderly people, pressure on natural resources, and a fear of over-population. This fear of over-population leads to pressure on people to have fewer children, and in turn this leads to social conflicts over the right to bear children. This social conflict is already apparent in our society (see Chapter Four of this book). Slaughter's paper is worth reading in its entirety, and is No. 5 of an occasional series of papers from the Centre for Peace Studies, St Martin's College, Lancaster.

11 The Chinese government has had a policy of encouraging the population to be satisfied with smaller families for some time now. An account of ways in which population control has worked out in practice over the last ten to fifteen years will be found in *Women and Childcare in China: A Firsthand Report*, by Ruth Sidel, Penguin, 1982. The difficulties being caused through the operation of the very recent policy designed to limit the fertile population to one child per family are described in an article by Elisabeth Croll, 'China's first-born nightmare returns', *The Guardian*, 28 October 1983. There was also a BBC 2 *Horizon* television programme on this topic on 7 November 1983.

The relationship between population control and economic development is an area of some controversy. Like many economists, Todaro, *op. cit.*, considers that population control policies are not a major factor in development. He feels that development of itself will lead to a natural fall in the birthrate. However, others, like L. R. Brown, in *Population Policies for a New Economic Era*, Worldwatch Institute, Washington, 1983, believe that population increases prevent economic growth.

12 The Prime Minister of Singapore, Lee Kwan Yew, made an unscripted National Day Speech, in August 1983, on his fears of an impending genetic collapse of the population of Singapore, unless the better-educated women could be persuaded to have more children. The problem had arisen because two-thirds of male graduates were marrying beneath their educational level, and many female graduates remained unmarried. Using Professor Thomas Bouchard, Minnesota, as his authority, the Prime Minister supported the 'nature' side of the 'nature versus nurture' debate on the subject of human intelligence. According to Brian Eads of *The Observer*, 18 September 1983, many Singaporeans were blaming 'women's liberation' for this situation. In many ways this situation seems ironic, as in Singapore the population is being held down by an active campaign for a two-child family. And personal observation would suggest that 'nurture' has had an important effect on the upbringing of most Singaporeans, in that they are an industrious community, which sets a high value on educational achievement.

13 A survey by the Legal and General Insurance Company, commissioned from Gallup, showed that although having a child was likely to be a couple's most expensive investment, few were deterred from having children because of expense; and only 3 per cent of parents perceived no advantages to having children. 26 per cent of those interviewed thought children gave considerable pleasure, and 17 per cent thought children improved family life. The results of this survey were summarised in *The Times*, 23 September 1983.

14 Article 16(1) of the *Universal Declaration of Human Rights* states that men and women of full age, without any limitation due to race, nationality or religion, have the right to marry and to found a family.

15 As was stated in Chapter Two, the percentage of the population estimated to be childless is between about 10 and 15 per cent. In these circumstances, women of childbearing age need to have, on average, 2.2–2.3 children, in order to allow for their own replacement, and to replace the population lost by those who do not have children. A zero population growth rate is achieved when the number of live births falls below the replacement rate among fertile women (although immigration of children may affect the situation).

16 A MORI/*Sunday Times* poll, discussed in the *Sunday Times* on 6 November 1983, showed that 50 per cent of the public interviewed would make defence a priority for any cuts in government spending, whereas only 12 per cent would make it a priority for increases. In contrast, 4 per cent would make the National Health Service a priority for cuts in spending, as against 59 per cent who believe there should be an increase in NHS funding. A further poll, a week later, (*Sunday Times*, 13 November 1983), showed that a large majority of those interviewed felt that NHS cuts could not be made without harming the health service, and causing added suffering to patients.

The Brandt Report (*North–South: A Programme for Survival*, Pan, 1980) shows that the build-up of arms, particularly in the Third World, leads to growing instability and undermines development. 'The world's military spending dwarfs any spending on development' (p. 117). Also, the Council on Economic Priorities reported that high military spending affected the real growth in GDP, even in the more affluent countries. Between 1960 and 1979, the annual average rate of real growth in GDP was just over 3 per cent in the United States, while military spending as a percentage of GDP was nearly 8 per cent. Japan, by contrast, has a real growth rate of nearly 9 per cent, against military spending of about 1 per cent (these figures and others are summarised in the handbook to *Utopia Limited*, International Broadcasting Trust, 1983, which accompanied a series of programmes about world development issues on Channel Four television, Autumn 1983).

Chapter Six

1 Garrey *et al.*, *op. cit.*, p. 400.
2 Philipp and Carruthers, *op. cit.*, p. 6.

Chapter Seven

1 The birth statistics for 1984 show that there were 637,700 live births in England and Wales, and 135,200 abortions. These figures are provisional. Source: *Population Trends*, 44, Summer 1986, Office of Population Censuses and Surveys.

2 For the actual figures on babies and children adopted each year by non-relatives, see ch. 10, Note 1.

3 Statistics suggest that about 47 per cent of single parents (mostly women) are dependent on state benefits as their main source of income (see the summarised report on the Conference on the Family, held by the British Association for

Population Studies, published in *The Guardian*, 17 September 1983, under the title 'Conference on family supports plan to end divorce time limit'). Frank Field, MP in 'A poor show in the poverty war', *The Times*, 3 November 1983, states that in 1981 there were 370,000 single parents on welfare, caring for 620,000 children.

Despite the existence of poverty among one-parent families, many one-parent families manage to cope with their situation, and some single parents prefer to be on their own, rather than being locked into an unhappy relationship with a partner (see 'The truth is that today men need wives far more than women need husbands', Lynne Segal, *The Guardian*, 24 May 1983; also 'And baby makes two', Linda Taylor, *Observer*, 16 October 1983). Diana Davenport, *One Parent Families: A Practical Guide to Coping*, Pan, 1979, is a useful book for anyone who has to bring up children without the support of a partner.

4   For an account of the poverty and destitution that led a woman coping on her own to put her children in a Dr Barnardo's home before the last war, see Kathleen Dayus, *Her People*, Virago, 1982, Ch. 16. There are still people living who were brought up in the Workhouse, as a result of the destitution of their only parent.

5   Quoted in *Family Circle*, 13 July 1983, p. 28.

6   Desmond Morris, *The Book of Ages*, Cape, 1983, suggests that there is a difference between the ideal age for being pregnant, and the ideal age for being a mother. A 22 year-old woman has the smallest chance of losing her unborn child, but 27 is the age when a woman is least likely to suffer the death of her newborn baby. The fecundity of the 22 year-old is not matched by her experience of giving birth, while the 27 year-old is superior in producing live babies because there is a greater chance that her system has been through pregnancy before.

7   Elisabeth Badinter, *The Myth of Motherhood: An Historical View of the Maternal Instinct*, Souvenir Press, 1981, p. 327. This topic is also dealt with in Lee Comer, *Wedlocked Women*, Feminist Books, 1974. She suggests that the social conditioning which leads women to see motherhood as the activity that completes and confirms their feminine identity is harmful to women; and in the way it works in our society it does not necessarily benefit children. Lynne Segal (ed)), *What is to be done about the Family?*, Penguin Books/The Socialist Society, 1983, contains articles on the theory and development of feminist thinking in relation to the family and motherhood. See particularly the articles by Mica Nava and Susan Himmelweit. Articles in Elizabeth Whitelegg, (ed) *et al.*, *The Changing Experience of Women*, Martin Robertson/The Open University, 1982 may be found useful; in particular those by Felicity Edholm and Adrienne Rich. The latter's article comes from her book *Of Woman Born: Motherhood as Experience & Institution*, Virago, 1977. This is a moving account of the conflict between selflessness and self-realisation that becomes a necessary condition of motherhood under present social, economic and political arrangements. There are also useful articles by Nancy Chodorov and Suan Contratto, and by Sara Ruddick in *Rethinking the Family: Some Feminist Questions*, edited by Barry Thorn with Marilyn Yalom, Longman, 1982.

Two general points that emerge from consideration of the above are: fatherhood is somehow belittled in the concentration on the importance of motherhood; and the necessity for strong mother-child bonding in the first years of a child's life is not a universal fact (other societies have different arrangements).

8   See Owens, *op. cit.*

9   Pfeffer and Woollett, *op. cit.*, p. 1. Also Marge Berer, 'Infertility – a suitable case for treatment?', *Marxism Today*, June 1985, argues for a more positive approach to infertility within a socialist feminist perspective.

10   See Segal (ed.), *op. cit.*, p. 217. It is interesting that feminist literature, and anthropological and sociological studies of women in the Third World, take the need for a woman to have access to fertility controls as a given; there is virtually

nothing written about the position of an infertile woman in the societies studied. Yet because of the complex of factors which force women in many societies to see motherhood as their only road to achievement, esteem and self-respect, one would have thought that the lives of women who do not achieve motherhood would be found more worthy of consideration in the literature.

Chapter Eight

1   Colin Murray-Parkes, *Bereavement: Studies of Grief in Adult Life*, Penguin, 1986, p. 202. The whole of Chap. 11, 'Reactions to other types of loss' is worth reading.

Chapter Nine

1   1 Corinthians, Chapter 13, verses 4–7, New International Version of the Bible.
2   The marriage and divorce figures for 1984 are as follows:

MALES:	Numbers (in thousands)
First marriages	255.5
Remarriages	81.4
FEMALES:	
First marriages	260.4
Remarriages	76.9
DIVORCES:	
Decrees absolute	144.5

Thus there were about 337,000 marriages and about 144,500 divorces. This works out at about one divorce for every 2.3 marriages.
3   This point is discussed in more detail in the following chapter.
4   See the discussion on myths about childlessness, Chapter Five.
5   Although this assumption lies behind much of the literature on the family as a social system, it is recognised that it is difficult to define what these ties, duties and dependencies are. The point is made by Robert and Rhona Rapoport, that:

> families in Britain today are in a transition from coping in a society in which there was a single overriding norm of what family life should be like to a society in which a plurality of norms are recognised as legitimate and, indeed, desirable. ('British families in transition', in *Families in Britain*, edited by R. N. Rapoport *op. cit.*, Routledge & Kegan Paul, 1982, p. 476).

6   Who is, and who is not, an important member of the family by virtue of his or her relationship to other family members, is difficult to decide objectively. Sociologists appear to accept that the inner nuclear core of parent(s) and children is one definite feature of the family. But beyond this, individual subjective perceptions of who is, and who is not, 'close kin', seem to be the main determinants in assigning importance to family roles (see D. H. J. Morgan, 'The social definition of the family', in *Sociology of the Family*, edited by Michael Anderson, Penguin, 1980). Michael Fogarty and Barbara Rodgers, in 'Family policy – international perspectives' (Rapoport, ed., *op. cit.*) show how grandparents tend to be seen to be outside the 'family' when issues of social policy are considered. They suggest that policymakers should aim to include the extended family within their terms of reference; also that in many communities grandparents have more influence in family life than is recognised by policymakers. Correspondence in the files of the National Association for the Childless would suggest that for many of the childless the role of grandparent is subjectively perceived to be an important role.
7   Why the concept of the family should have remained viable, when so many influences have combined to produce changes in the nature and function of the

family, is not an easy question to answer. A useful place to start would be 'Conventional families' by Ann Oakley, in Rapoport *et al.*, (eds), *op. cit.* Another interesting article is 'Is there a family? New anthropological views', by Jane Collier *et al.*, in Thorne and Yalom, (eds), *op. cit.* Lynne Segal, 'The most important thing of all – rethinking the family: an overview', in Segal, ed., *op. cit.*, makes the point that the traditional model of the family remains central to all family ideology, but it no longer corresponds to the typical household unit. Felicity Edholm, 'The unnatural family', in Whitelegg *et al.*, *op. cit.*, questions the universality of the notion of family as understood in contemporary Western society.

8   See the discussion on donor insemination in Chapter Four (p. 35), in particular the results of a NAC survey on attitudes to AID (Owens, *op. cit.*). In-vitro fertilisation, also, if developed further, has the potential to help many more infertile couples (see p. 37). These represent ways of having a 'child of one's own' that may seem preferable to adoption. As to reasons why alternative forms of nurture are not generally seen as a solution to childlessness, it has been suggested that for most people, having children is regarded as a very important experience in life (see Chapter Five). Why the childless do not readily come to see the advantages of the childfree life-style (Chapter Two); and why many childless women, in particular, do not see themselves to be 'liberated' from the need to find fulfilment in society by becoming a mother, as a result of an understanding of the feminist viewpoint; these are very interesting and important questions. They are, however, beyond the scope of the present book.

9   The whole area of male–female relationships in societies which admit of a distinction between a child born legitimately, and one born illegitimately, is very complex, and illegitimacy is generally very little documented. There seem to be countries and societies which discourage illegitimate births; but once the child is born, steps are taken to regularise the child's status, or to ensure that the child does not suffer any undue stigma or deprivation (see C. C. Zimmerman, 'The Atomistic Family', in Anderson, ed., *op. cit.*, also Gail W. Lapidus, *Women in Soviet Society: Equality, Development and Social Change*, University of California Press, 1978).

There are, conversely, countries and societies where the birth of an illegitimate child has such traumatic consequences for the families involved (or, more often, the woman's family) that the whole area of illegitimacy becomes 'taboo', and it is very difficult to find out much about how it is handled within one of these societies. We were told by a student from the Abadan area of Southern Iran of a case where a girl had been raped, and the man involved was taken to court by the authorities. The girl's brothers, however, killed her in the courtroom because of the shame and dishonour she had brought upon her family. It would appear that the social sanctions operating to prevent pre-marital intercourse on the part of the woman, make it unlikely that single women would willingly permit themselves to take part in a sexual relationship outside marriage. It would appear to be even less likely that such a woman would give birth to an illegitimate child. The fate of the young single girl who becomes pregnant is described by Nawal El Saadawi (*The Hidden Face of Eve: Women in the Arab World*, Zed Press, 1980):

[She] becomes in the eyes of society an unmarried woman, pregnant with child, or in other words a fallen depraved girl, devoid of virtue or honour. She faces the world alone and her life may terminate in suicide or in a murder committed by her father or another male member of the family. Alternatively she may die during an abortion carried out by one of the primitive rural methods resorted to despite its dangers. If she survives the abortion, she is liable to be prosecuted legally since abortion is not permitted by the law, and if she has to bring up her child, life becomes an interminable, long drawn out source of humiliation and misery.

An illegitimate girl child in a poor society like the one above, has very little chance of leading any kind of reasonable life. Why social controls on fertility exist, and how they operate to further or limit the contribution of particular societies to the gene pool of the future, is an area that has been very little studied.

10 We know of more than one instance among the immigrant community of the Midlands, where a marriage has broken down because of the husband's infertility; yet divorce has seemed preferable, rather than the husband having to admit his infertility by seeking medical treatment.

Lois Beck and Nikki Keddie (eds), *Women in the Muslim World*, Harvard University Press, 1978, contains several articles on the importance of having children in the assessment of a married woman's social status. Articles by Nancy Tapper and Caroll Pastner describe societies where the wife's proven or assumed infertility is a *prima facie* reason for the husband to divorce her. However, the Quran does not contain any specific reference to infertility as constituting a reason for divorce (see *The Meaning of the Glorious Koran*, by Mohammed Marmaduke Pickthall, Mentor, n.d.). El Saadawi, *op. cit.*, has a chapter on marriage and divorce in Arab countries, and Nadia Youssef, in Beck and Keddie, *op. cit.*, discusses the status of pronatalism in Islamic doctrine.

11 The currently held philosophy behind the medical research into, and the treatment of, infertility would seem to imply that infertility is largely seen as some kind of 'mechanical' breakdown in the physical structure of the organs involved in reproduction; or as the failure of some chemical message originating with the glandular and/or hormonal systems of the body. In the terms of this philosophy, medical science would appear to have been highly successful in attributing most causes of infertility to one of the two major categories above. This would appear to leave very little room for manoeuvre for any contending genetic explanation, except in fairly rare instances.

12 Richard Dawkins, *The Selfish Gene*, Paladin, 1978, talks about evolution by non-genetic means (ch. 11). He posits the existence of a new replicator, a unit of cultural transmission called a *meme*, unique to humans, which is already achieving a rate of evolutionary change which has outpaced that of the gene. Much of the current technology, and scientific and social change, is a result of propagation of memes in the meme pool, 'leaping from brain to brain via a process which, in the broad sense, can be called imitation' (p. 206). Dawkins develops this idea rather tentatively, and it is as yet somewhat speculative. However, in the following paragraphs of this present chapter of our book we wish to acknowledge the influence of his conception of the cultural meme in our assessment of the possibilities open to the childless, in becoming contributors to the future of the society in which they live.

Chapter Ten

1

	1975	1980	1983	1984
Total adoptions in England and Wales	21,299	10,609	9,029	7,945
Joint adoptions (one adopter is parent of the child)	9,262	3,668	2,972	4,195
Children adopted by non-relatives	12,037	6,941	6,057	3,750

These figures do not discriminate between adoptions of babies and older children. Thus the actual figures for the adoption of babies and very young children are likely to be somewhat less than the figures given for numbers of children adopted by non-relative couples. In particular, the size of the drop between 1983 and 1984 should be noted. The figures are taken from *The Children Act 1975: Second Report to Parliament*, House of Commons, 21 November 1984, HMSO.

2   There has been no research to test the hypothesis that a couple adopting a child during their fertile years are likely to have their own natural child subsequently. To substantiate this view would require a study of those who had adopted and who had subsequently given birth to a natural child; and a comparison made between their fertility, and that of others in their age group. Only if it could be established that those within the age group were *more* likely to give birth after adopting could the myth be established as a fact. As some adopters are infertile before they adopt, they could not be part of such a sample, and only those with unexplained infertility or borderline infertility could be affected. There is nothing to show that such people conceive more than others in the same age group.

There are two possible reasons for the persistence of the myth. The first is historical: in earlier periods fertile people often adopted children. Almost inevitably they would have their own natural children as well. Also, it is not only the infertile who adopt at the present time. Secondly, a few people with fertility problems do become pregnant without medical help; thus when they conceive after adoption there is a tendency to relate the conception to the prior adoption. Since infertility is mainly a medical problem, adoption and fertility are unlikely to be linked. It is hard to see how the one could affect the other, except, perhaps, that the tension and stress between the couple may be believed to be lowered as a result of the adoption. There is, however, no evidence to bear out this belief.

3   There are no statistics or research which reliably show how many people are enquiring about adoption. A generally accepted but unsatisfactory way to calculate how many people might be enquiring at any one time is to take as a basic assumption the figures of one in six couples needing help with infertility treatment (about 1,500,000 couples). Of these, in any one year 300,000 individuals or couples are thought to be having some form of medical investigation. The National Association for the Childless estimates that about a third of couples undergoing or ending treatment unsuccessfully enquire about adoption. This would suggest that there are about 100,000 couples pursuing the roughly 4,000 babies and children available for adoption by 'strangers' each year.

4   See the estimates in note 3 above.

5   The background to this is described in C. R. Smith, *Adoption and Fostering: Why and How*, Macmillan, 1984, chapter 1; also B. Jordan, *Invitation to Social Work*, Basil Blackwell, 1984, pp. 17–18, 144, 176; N. Parton, *The Politics of Child Abuse*, Macmillan, 1985, chapters 5, 7, 8. Parton, in particular, is against frequent use of adoption in childcare practice.

Putting the case for adoption are B. Tizard, *Adoption: A Second Chance*, Open Books, 1977, and J. Goldstein, A. Freud and A. J. Solnit, *Beyond the Best Interests of the Child*, Burnett Books, 1980.

6   The arguments for and against transracial adoption are given in: R. J. Simon and H. Altstein, *Transracial Adoption: A Follow-Up*, Lexington Books, 1981; O. Gill and B. Jackson, *Adoption and Race*, Batsford, St Martins Press and British Agencies for Adoption and Fostering, 1983.

What little research has been done into this area suggests that most transracial adoptions compare favourably with same-race adoptions. However, in terms of racial identity, the children studied seemed to be being brought up as 'white in all but skin colour and had little knowledge or experience of their counterparts growing up in the black community' (Gill and Jackson, p. 130). However, it is stressed by all the researchers that the children studied were comparatively young at the time of the study, and that it will have to be seen how the children experience their racial identity as independent adults.

7   The British Agencies for Adoption and Fostering have issued a Statement of Policy on Inter-Country Adoption (dated February 1986) and are involved in discussions with the Home Office and Department of Health and Social Security at the time of

going to press. The major concerns are the way children are brought into the country without prior official clearance, the many forms of abuse surrounding the adoption of children from overseas, and the possible failure of the private adopters to appreciate the implications of bringing up a child from overseas. It is difficult to know how effectively some of the suggestions for controls can be implemented.

8 See Tizard, *op. cit.*, Gill and Jackson, *op. cit.*, C. R. Smith, 1984, *op. cit.*
9 The requirements for would-be adopters are spelt out in *Adopting a Child*, British Agencies for Adoption and Fostering, (1984–5 edition).
10 See *Adopting a Child* (note 9). It is sometimes possible for single people to be considered for the more specialist adoption and fostering tasks.
11 See note 7.
12 See *Adopting a Child* (note 9).
13 *Adopting a Child*, p. 18.
14 *Adopting a Child*, p. 18.
15 C. R. Smith, *Adoption Policy and Practice*, Ph.D. thesis, University of Leeds, 1980. Referred to in C. R. Smith, 1984, *op. cit.*, p. 83.
16 See. D. Renne, 'There's always adoption', *Child Welfare*, 56 (1977), pp. 465–70. The practice described relates to the United States context.
17 The principles and practice of this approach are described in C. R. Smith, 1984, *op. cit.*, (chapter 5 in particular).
18 Muriel Dimen, 'Towards the Reconstruction of Sexuality' (forthcoming). Quoted in A. M. Jaggar, *Feminist Politics and Human Nature*, Harvester Press, 1983, p. 389.

Chapter Eleven

1 Pfeffer and Woollett, *op. cit.*, pp. 12–13.
2 See Pfeffer and Woollett, *op. cit.*, and Eck Menning, *op. cit.*

Chapter Twelve

1 Pfeffer and Woollett, *op. cit.*, p. 13.
2 The National Association for the Childless is very willing to send details of help available by them and through different organisations, for those suffering as a result of traumatic experiences and conditions connected with infertility. The three books in the selected reading list on miscarriage, stillbirth and infant death may be helpful to some. There is also a support organisation, The Stillbirth and Neonatal Society (SANDS). NAC has a leaflet on hysterectomy and the young woman, by Barbara Eck Menning, reproduced by permission of RESOLVE; and a hysterectomy support group has been set up by Judy Vaughan. For further information on the above, please write to NAC.
Pfeffer and Woollett, *op. cit.*, contains a list of useful addresses for those suffering from several conditions associated with infertility.
3 Quoted from 'A positive approach' by Annette Garland, *The Times*, 17 August 1983.
4 From 'Women dogged by despond', Veronica Horwell, *The Sunday Times*, 10 July 1983. It is interesting to note that 74 per cent of people requesting information on depression, as a result of the Channel Four television series *Well Being*, were women. See *Well being: an evaluation*, by R. McCron and E. Dean, Broadcasting Support Services, 1983.
5 See Peter Parrish, *Medicines: A Guide for Everybody*, Penguin, 1982. This is an easy-to-read reference book that does not require any specialist knowledge to understand. Although it has been revised four times since its first publication in 1976, and is fairly comprehensive, it may not always include the very latest drugs available. As some of these very new drugs sometimes appear to have nasty side-effects which are reported and discussed in the national press, anyone put on one of

these drugs should enquire of their doctor what kind of risks may be involved in taking them.

R. B. Fisher and G. A. Christie, *A Dictionary of Drugs*, Paladin, 1982. This book deals with the major drug groups under separate headings, and requires some knowledge of chemistry and physiology to obtain maximum use from it. It is, however, most useful in giving information about the history of a drug, its major uses, and known side effects.

Another useful source is E. Trimmer, *Good Housekeeping Guide to Medicines*, Ebury Press, 1983.

The problems connected with addiction to tranquillisers, sedatives and sleeping pills are discussed in the *Annual Report 1982–3* of the Medical Research Council.

6   See Parrish, *op. cit.*, p. 75.

7   *St Matthew*, 7, 27, Authorised Version of the Bible.

8   See Eck Menning, *op. cit.*, chaps 13 and 14. also Pfeffer and Woollett, *op. cit.*, ch. 10.

9   'Ronald Searle – pursued by the curse of St Trinian's', interview by Philip Norman, *The Sunday Times*, 17 October 1982.

Chapter Thirteen

1   It is interesting that John Nicholson, who supervised the Colchester Survey on Ageing, found that there were three different types of 'active' approach to old age. People could pursue activities which made no concessions to old age; or hobbies and interests which were more appropriate for the retired; or they could invest in people rather than activities, and become the hub of a network of friends and relatives. These responses do not seem very different from those described in this chapter of the present book. See the chapter 'Life after work', in John Nicholson, *Seven Ages*, Fontana, 1980.

2   This quotation comes from a conversation between Lord Goodman and Miriam Gross, which was recorded for the occasion of Lord Goodman's 70th birthday, in the *Observer* of 21 August 1983. Miriam Gross had asked him whether he regretted not having had children. The whole interview is worth reading to see that being childless is only one aspect of a life that is seen in many ways as having been full of interest, achievement and challenge.

Chapter Fourteen

1   A. J. P. Taylor, *A Personal History*, Atheneum, 1983.

2   Elaine Evans was interviewed in a Granada television programme in the *World in Action* series, under the title of 'A Widow's Story'. This was screened on the 15 August 1983, and the particular quotation was reproduced in a review of the programme by Mick Brown in *The Guardian* which appeared the following day.

Suggested Reading

1 INFERTILITY

Barbara Eck Menning, *Infertility: A Guide for the Childless Couple*, Prentice-Hall, 1977.
A helpful, wide-ranging account of the medical and psychological aspects of infertility, written by an American nurse specialist who has been through experience of infertility herself. She founded the American support organisation for the infertile, RESOLVE. Unfortunately, the book is out of print, but it might be available through libraries.

Naomi Pfeffer and Anne Woollett, *The Experience of Infertility*, Virago, 1983.
A comprehensive and stimulating account of infertility, written from the feminist point of view, by two women who have experienced infertility. The medical aspects are well-described and illustrated, and there is much valuable information about the feelings of women who have experienced infertility. There are detailed notes, a useful annotated reading list, and information on organisations dealing with infertility and related problems.

Elliot E. Philipp and G. Barry Carruthers (eds), *Infertility*, William Heinemann, 1981.
A textbook for professionals, containing a variety of articles on all medical aspects of infertility. It is based on the work of the Royal Northern Hospital Philip Hill Parenthood Clinic, and shows the importance of a team approach to infertility investigation and treatment. A fair amount of medical knowledge is required to make use of the book, but it is a most valuable guide to current medical practice in good fertility clinics and departments.

John J. Stangel, *Fertility & Conception*, Paddington Press, 1979.
A very detailed account of the medical aspects of infertility by an American doctor. It would make a useful reference book for anyone undergoing infertility investigations. There is a glossary of medical terms, and the book is well-illustrated. Unfortunately, out of print, but it may be available through libraries.

Dr Anna M. Flynn and Melissa Brooks, *A Manual of Natural Family Planning*, George Allen & Unwin, 1984.
This well-written book will be of use to those who wish to increase their fertility awareness through natural observations. A most helpful book for women who wish to understand fully their monthly fertility cycle.

Robert and Elizabeth Snowden, *The Gift of a Child*, George Allen & Unwin, 1984.
A most informative book on all aspects of artificial insemination by donor (AID). Essential reading for anyone contemplating undertaking donor insemination.

Andrew Stanway, *Why Us? A Commonsense Guide for the Childless*, Thorsons, 1984.
A popular, fairly easy-to-read account of infertility, written by a doctor and medical journalist. A sympathetic introduction to the topic.

2   MISCARRIAGE, STILLBIRTH AND INFANT DEATH

Susan Borg and Judith Lasker, *When Pregnancy Fails: Coping with Miscarriage, Stillbirth & Infant Death*, Routledge & Kegan Paul, 1982.
A book to help those who have suffered a miscarriage, stillbirth or infant death to grieve and mourn for their lost child, to come to terms with their loss, and to begin to hope again. It is written by two American women who each lost their own child at, or shortly after, birth. It contains extensive references, a glossary, and lists of useful organisations and resources.

Hank Pizer and Christine O'Brien Palinski, *Coping with a Miscarriage*, Jill Norman, 1980.
An account of the medical, genetic and emotional aspects of miscarriage. Each chapter contains a concluding summary of its main points. A practical and useful book, based on the personal experience of one of the writers, and the medical knowledge of the other. It contains references, and a glossary.

Ann Oakley, Ann McPherson and Helen Roberts, *Miscarriage*, Fontana Paperbacks, 1984.
A most sympathetic, helpful and informative book. Essential reading on all aspects of miscarriage.

3   ADOPTION

Adopting a Child: A Brief Guide for Prospective Adopters, British Agencies for Adoption and Fostering, 1984–5.
A short booklet, containing basic information on how to become an adoptive parent. It describes the relevant regulations and selection procedures. The adoption agencies operating in England, Scotland and Wales are listed, together with their regulations and preferences. There is also a booklist. The booklet stresses that there are very few babies available for adoption, that selection procedures are rigorous, and that many adoption agencies may close their lists from time to time.

Jane Rowe, *Yours by Choice: A Guide for Adoptive Parents*, Routledge & Kegan Paul, new edition 1982.
Essential reading for any couple who are considering whether they should apply to adopt. It is clearly written, and gives important advice as to the questions that a couple should ask themselves, to ensure that they understand their own motives, and that they would be able to cope with a child who was not born to them. It stresses that most children available for adoption will have special problems or needs. A comprehensive and useful book; also easy to read.

Index

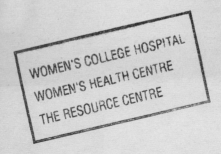